Childhood Illness and the Allergy Connection

Childhood Illness and the Allergy Connection

A Nutritional Approach to Overcoming and Preventing Childhood Illness

Zoltan P. Rona, M.D.

PRIMA PUBLISHING

Publisher and Author believe the information contained in this book to be reliable and accurate at the time of publication. However, because of the constant changes in medical science, Publisher and Author must disclaim any warranty that the information is accurate or complete. Moreover, this book is not intended to be a substitute for professional medical advice. Readers should consult a physician or other medical professional for the proper diagnosis and treatment of childhood illness and allergies. The reader assumes all liability or responsibility for any damage or loss, whether indirect or direct, caused by any use of the information contained in this book.

PRIMA PUBLISHING and colophon are registered trademarks of Prima Communications, Inc.

Library of Congress Cataloging-in-Publication Data

Rona, Zoltan P., 1951—
   Childhood illness and the allergy connection: a nutritional approach to overcoming and preventing childhood illness / Zoltan Rona.
       p.   cm.
   Includes bibliographical references and index.
   ISBN 0-7615-0611-X
   1. Allergy in children—Nutritional aspects.   2. Allergy in children—Complications.   I. Title.
RJ399.A4R66   1996
618.92'970654—dc20   96-31761
                                        DEC 1 8 1996   CIP

96 97 98 99 HH 10 9 8 7 6 5 4 3 2 1
Printed in the United States of America

How to Order:
Single copies may be ordered from Prima Publishing, P.O. Box 1260BK, Rocklin, CA 95677; telephone (916) 632-4400. Quantity discounts are also available. On your letterhead, include information concerning the intended use of the books and the number of books you wish to purchase.

Visit us online at http://www.primapublishing.com

Lovingly dedicated to my wife, Sharon, and our
two sons, Matthew and Darcy

Contents

Acknowledgments

The following people deserve credit for their inspiration, suggestions, help, and support in making this book possible:

Sharon E. Rona, my wife, who has always stood by my side and helped me understand a great deal about childhood issues which weren't medical or nutritional.

Dr. Norbert Kerenyi, a lifelong friend, for his help in so many areas, as well as for his terrific sense of humor.

Dr. Vivien Smith, a constant source of wisdom and kind support in helping me shed light on psychosocial childhood issues.

My secretarial and office support staff: Kristine Drasutis, Jessica and Ihor Borowets, Emma Lindops, and Chris Wowk, who have all helped make my office work a great deal more pleasant and less stressful.

Dr. Robert Sager, a good friend and colleague with a rare understanding of both conventional medicine and its alternatives.

Mr. David Wolf, the world's best accountant, for his invaluable help and advice.

All the Children of the Holocaust who are themselves now looking for more gentle health care for their own children.

All of my private practice patients who encouraged me to write this book.

Introduction

The information contained in this book is not a replacement for orthodox care in any area of diagnosis or treatment. Rather, it is a supplement to it. When it comes to chronic illnesses of childhood, conventional methods of prescription drugs and surgery are by no means the only effective treatments.

While I fully acknowledge that the family doctor and pediatrician are able to help children with allergy-related problems using conventional therapies, there are many children who benefit more from an alternative approach. This book was written primarily to inform parents of alternative approaches to childhood illnesses and what may be some of the underlying causes of them and the role of allergies in causing or worsening them. I believe that no one therapy suits all. This book will help parents and children understand both therapeutic philosophies while giving practical tips on prevention.

"Nonconventional" Approaches to Treatment of Allergies

"Alternative" and "complementary" are two terms used interchangeably to describe a type of medical practice which involves the patient more actively in his or her own medical care. Alternative medicine is consistent with the principles of the great founders of medicine, such as Hippocrates with his oath embracing the principle "above all, do no harm." Alternative medicine primarily makes use of natural substances, but its wisest practitioners use the best of conventional medical drugs and surgery along with natural therapies such as herbs, acupuncture, and homeopathy. For this reason, the term "complementary medicine," coined by British doctors to describe this more inclusive approach, might be more suitable.

My strong interest in medical alternatives started with a curiosity about natural ways to improve my skills and stamina as a tournament tennis player. When I took vitamin and mineral supplements, I saw the results in my improved performance on the tennis court. I had hoped that my medical training would provide information on nutrition. To my disappointment, medical school provided no instruction at all in this field. The best nutritional information existed in medical libraries, but none of it was ever presented in any organized way to the students. Schools of naturopathy and chiropractic and other sources of information on natural therapies were either ignored or attacked by my medical professors.

I turned to complementary medicine shortly after graduation despite the opposition of my peers. Why? Partly because of my own interest and partially because of the high public demand for information on diet and supplemental nutrients. In the late 1970s, when I began practicing medicine, there already existed the beginnings of an attitude shift toward natural alternatives. My training in conventional medicine was simply not enough to deal with what a growing segment of the public was demanding.

My evolution from mainstream medical practice was a gradual process lasting over a decade. I took special training in medical alternatives, including a four-year master's degree program in biochemistry and clinical nutrition. I also attended various seminars and courses for naturopathic doctors and traveled often to learn what I could about complementary medicine.

Part of this process for me involved the loss of my blind faith in some of the dogma of medical orthodoxy which claimed, among other things, that nutrition had nothing to do with the cause of chronic disease. Despite a great deal of evidence to the contrary, especially in the past decade, the notion that diet and lifestyle are not important factors in disease is still often entrenched in medical orthodoxy. Taking off the blinders did not leave me with less respect for my conventional medical colleagues. It just meant that my allegiance shifted more toward my patients, who had lived with the consequences of a narrow-minded approach and wanted more.

Mainstream medicine leaves a lot to be desired in the treatment or prevention of chronic childhood illnesses such as asthma, recurrent middle-ear infections, hyperactivity, and behavioral disorders. At best, conventional medicine suppresses the symptoms. At worst, it creates new diseases, iatrogenic diseases, or further harms and sometimes even kills its clients through the side effects of drugs and surgery. Adverse reactions to "safe and effective" prescription drugs cause nearly 200,000 deaths, send nine million people to the hospital, and cost the United States more than $76 billion annually. In addition, conventional medicine does virtually nothing to address the sources of disease: stress, bad diets, and dangerous lifestyles.

The Growth of Complementary Medicine

The desire to overcome chronic diseases that respond poorly to conventional medicine is a major cause of the recent surge in interest in medical alternatives. But there are other causes. One obvious cause is the growing number of immigrants coming to North America from parts of the world where herbs, vitamins, massage therapy, homeopathy, and spa therapies are highly respected. Excellent examples of such groups are the Chinese (traditional Chinese medicine and acupuncture), East Indians (Ayurvedic medicine), and Eastern Europeans (herbs and spa treatments such as hydrotherapy).

How Do Conventional Medicine and Complementary Medicine Differ?

There are two important issues to be considered in understanding the basic differences between conventional and complementary healing practices: time and healing philosophy. Most children and their parents have experienced the "one in, one out" approach of the average pediatrician or family doctor. In Toronto, where I practice, it is not unusual for a conventional medical practitioner to see over one hundred children in an eight-hour day. Some specialists have been documented to see over two hundred children per day. These brief encounters, for the most part, do not easily lend themselves to anything but a quick fix via a prescription drug. The natural health care practitioner, who rarely sees more than a dozen clients a day, creates the time to focus on education: helping children and their parents to find out why they got ill and what they can do on a daily basis to prevent their illnesses. Comlementary practitioners encourage self-care and self-responsibility.

Complementary practitioners demand more from their clients in terms of lifestyle and diet changes. They involve clients in an educative process, and this takes a great deal of time. It means becoming a partner in the process with the doctor. It means doing a lot of reading, exploring, and trial and error. For many, this is empowering—a welcome change from the doctor's office where the client's medical records are secret and the sole property of the medical practitioner. But this process is not for everyone, especially for those interested in a "quick fix." Complementary medicine is for clients who want to take more control over their health and who are willing to follow through on their responsibility once they've taken the reins.

A good example of the different approaches of a conventional and a complementary doctor can be found in the treatment of recurrent ear infections in children. The conventional treatment involves repetitive prescriptions for broad-spectrum antibiotics and, in the most resistive cases, the surgical implantation of plastic tubes into the middle ear to provide continuous drainage. Treatment depends entirely upon drugs and/or surgery—a simple matter of swallowing pills and/or lying anesthetized in the operating room. A natural health care practitioner, on the other hand, would advise the elimination of sugar, refined carbohydrates, milk, and other potential food allergy triggers or suppressors of the immune system. He or she may also recommend a friendly bacterial culture such as *lactobacillus acidophilus,* herbs (echinacea, goldenseal, calendula, garlic, parsley, hypericum, and others), vitamins (A, B complex, and C), minerals (zinc, selenium), or other substances (colloidal silver, propolis). The process involves education about diet and food supplements and can be applied to both treatment and prevention. Successful implementation involves much more than just swallowing an antibiotic capsule, antihistamine, or decongestant a few times daily; it depends on a change in the eating habits of the child.

The Conventional Allergy System

- Focuses on the effects of environmental inhalants—pollen, dust, mites, and molds—as illness-triggering agents.
- Holds that food and chemical allergies are rare and are related to IgE, an antibody family that can be diagnosed through skin tests only; asserts that real childhood disease has nothing to do with other antibody families such as IgG.
- Concerns itself with how IgE-mediated allergy relates to asthma, eczema, and anaphylactic reactions.
- Rarely, if ever, suggests blood testing for food and chemical allergies because these are viewed as unimportant.
- Acknowledges drug allergies but limits testing to skin testing for drugs such as penicillin and patch testing for contact dermatitis.
- Prescribes treatments involving removal of offending inhalant irritants and prescription of drugs such as antihistamines and

corticosteroids, allergy serum injections, and various types of inhaled drug sprays.

• Does not acknowledge multiple chemical hypersensitivity disorders or food allergies and their association to hyperactivity, middle-ear infections, gastrointestinal disorders, autoimmune conditions, and other problems.

• Suggests either tranquilizers or psychiatric treatment for children suffering from chronic fatigue syndrome, hyperactivity, learning disabilities, autism, mood disorders, migraine headaches, or multiple chemical hypersensitivities.

• Does not acknowledge any connection between immune system impairment and the frequent use of antibiotics and vaccinations.

• Often vehemently opposes natural approaches, especially homeopathy, acupuncture, muscle testing, and nutritional supplements.

• Is supported and enforced by medical associations, the pharmaceutical industry, licensing boards, the Food and Drug Administration (FDA), dietitians, insurance companies, and bureaucrats.

• Frequently attacks freedom of choice in health care, especially with respect to diagnosis and treatment of food allergies and candida, as well as the practice of environmental medicine (formerly known as clinical ecology).

The Complementary Medicine Allergy System

• Focuses on the whole person, including diet, activity level, and environment, as well as psychological and emotional aspects.

• Acknowledges the role of food and chemical allergies in triggering numerous chronic illnesses.

• Uses many different allergy testing techniques including elimination-provocation, IgG-RAST (Radio-Allergo-Sorbent-Tests),

ELISA (Enzyme-Linked Immunosorbent Assay) tests, electro-acupuncture, pulse testing, and others.

- Evaluates levels of vitamins and minerals by using blood, urine, and hair tests.

- Investigates the impact of gut bacterial flora, digestive enzyme adequacy, absorption problems, leaky gut syndrome, and other biochemical conditions that predispose children to chronic illness.

- Frequently finds delayed food and chemical allergies to be aggravating factors in chronic illnesses, including asthma, eczema, autoimmune diseases, and recurrent infections.

- Makes use of treatments such as chemical and food avoidance, rotation diets, avoidance of drugs if possible, neutralization, the use of organic foods, detoxification programs, vitamin and mineral therapies, and herbal remedies.

- Addresses underlying fungal and parasitic infections.

- Acknowledges the fact that frequent use of antibiotics and vaccinations may have something to do with immune system impairment.

- Is usually opposed by medical associations, the pharmaceutical industry, licensing boards, the FDA, dietitians, insurance companies, and bureaucrats.

- Supports freedom of choice in health care.

Conventional and Complementary Medicine Together

Conventional and complementary medicine do not have to be mutually exclusive. One can still visit the family doctor for a yearly checkup or for emergency care and see a natural health care practitioner for advice on how to prevent infections. A child on medication for asthma can also follow a hypoallergenic rotation diet and take antioxidant vitamins, minerals, and herbs. The natural therapies—be they herbs, vitamins, homeopathic remedies, or special diets—are not "alternatives" to conventional medical prescriptions, but modalities that can help make conventional treatments more effective.

In Europe, complementary approaches are not only on the rise but are being integrated into conventional medical practices. A recent study by the *British Medical Journal* revealed some staggering numbers:

• In the Netherlands, forty-seven percent of medical doctors now use some form of complementary therapy.

• Forty-six percent of Germans now use some form of complementary medicine to treat their illnesses, while seventy-seven percent of all German pain clinics use acupuncture.

• In France, forty-nine percent of the population uses complementary therapies. The number of children using homeopathy in France grew from sixteen percent of the population in 1982 to thirty-six percent in 1992.

• In Belgium, eighty-four percent of all homeopathy and seventy-four percent of all acupuncture treatment is provided by conventional doctors.

• The use of homeopathic remedies is growing by twenty percent each year in Great Britain and thirty percent each year in Greece and Portugal.

These statistics indicate the popular "arrival" of complementary health care. They signal a huge change in the psyche of the population in favor of more involvement in their health care. The survival of complementary health care systems will be dependent on the will of individuals to take more responsibility for their own health while continuing to demand preventive health care measures.

1

Expanding the Traditional View of Childhood Allergies

Scientifically controlled clinical trials have shown that only ten to twenty percent of all procedures used in present-day medical practices are of benefit to patients. It was concluded that the vast majority of medical procedures now being utilized routinely by physicians are "unproven" when subjected to the same rigid standards these same orthodox physicians are demanding of alternative, nutritional practitioners.

—*U.S. Office of Technology Assessment*

Why You Should Read This Book

As parents we have always depended upon the knowledge and skill of the medical profession to guide and help us in providing for the health care needs of our children. Traditionally, most of us (myself included) have never questioned the validity of routine medical checkups, immunizations, antibiotics, and other drug prescriptions. Very few of us ever doubted the wisdom of routine surgeries for tonsils and adenoids and the implanting of tubes for recurrent middle-ear infections. The past decade, however, has led to a reassessment of the logic of these cherished dogmas. The general state of health of our children is deteriorating, with more and more children forced to use prescription medications.

When I first started general practice in 1978, childhood asthma, hay fever, hyperactivity, and eczema were relatively uncommon. I saw no children suffering from chronic fatigue syndrome (CFS) that prevented them from going to school. Parents brought their children to me for checkups and immunizations. Conventional medicine was usually effective in dealing with episodes of illness. In the late 1980s, however, I saw a growing number of children with chronic illnesses, recurrent infections, and other puzzling health conditions such as CFS, which was almost nonexistent a decade ago. There are increasing numbers of childhood AIDS, depression, and learning disabilities. Why is this happening and why is the conventional medical approach ineffective in both preventing and treating these evolving phenomena? Do parents and their children have any options?

The traditional doctor-patient relationship is changing dramatically. Many parents, scientists, and physicians like myself are questioning both the safety and efficacy of practices which are doing very little, if anything, to prevent chronic childhood illnesses. For example, many parents in the 1990s are concerned about the alarming rise in the use of drugs like methylphenidate (Ritalin) for attention deficit disorder (ADD). Once a rarity in children, it is now unusual for a class to be without half a dozen children medicated for ADD, dyslexia, learning disabilities, or asthma. Isn't there a way of dealing with these conditions without resorting to amphetamine-like drugs? Why is there a growing number of both medical and lay groups that question the safety and efficacy of childhood immunizations?

Of concern to both parents and a growing number of holistic physicians is the use of antibiotics which weaken immunity while having no impact on resistant strains of bacteria. Once considered the magic bullets of medical orthodoxy, the overuse of antibiotics for self-limiting infections like the flu has all but rendered these drugs useless.

Another situation that is becoming more common with children is the daily use of steroid inhalers, creams, and injections. The parents of children with asthma, eczema, or rhinitis worry about the long-term hazards of drugs previously used only in life-threatening conditions. Isn't there anything else that can be done?

Parents are not getting answers to these questions simply because the majority of the medical profession is unaware of the fact that all of these childhood illnesses have an allergy connection. An allergy can be defined as a sensitivity to some substance in the environment (an allergen). The allergen (for example, wheat, milk, or corn) may be harmless to some people but causes a bad reaction in others. The reason this occurs has to do with several factors, including heredity and the overall condition of the immune system. Poor diet, nutrient deficiencies, stress, emotional traumas, drug use, inadequate sleep, and infections are other factors that can affect the way a child reacts to a food or chemical. The allergic reaction could express itself as hay fever, asthma, hives, headache, hyperactivity, hypoglycemia, stomachache, depression, a learning disability, or an autoimmune disease, such as juvenile rheumatoid arthritis, diabetes, or chronic fatigue syndrome.

As you will read in this book, a food allergy is not just something that causes an immediate anaphylactic (Type I), life-threatening reaction. Despite the fact that a great deal of published research confirms that asthma, recurrent middle-ear infections, ADD, eczema, autoimmune diseases such as juvenile rheumatoid arthritis and diabetes can all be traced to undiagnosed or unsuspected allergies, the medical profession has been slow and reluctant to deal with these underlying causes of childhood illness.

The good news for parents is that a growing number of health care practitioners have accepted the allergy connection in children. There are tests which can determine delayed (Type II) allergies so that a change in diet and lifestyle can be made. Natural immune-boosting supplements will also help reverse or, at the very least, control the illnesses associated with allergies. In some children, drugs will become unnecessary. In others, drugs can be markedly reduced. An increasing amount of published research is proving this.

How is it that food allergies can cause middle-ear infections, bed-wetting, and asthma? If it's really true that ADD is related to food and chemical allergies, why do doctors not use this approach? What can be done if doctors refuse to test and treat the allergies? These and other questions are the subject of this book. The message of this book is not that conventional medical treatment should be abandoned and replaced by food allergy testing and treatment, but that conventional medical treatment should be complemented with an approach to childhood illness that is scientific, prevention-oriented, and natural. In order for this to become a reality for children, both parents and their doctors have to have a deeper understanding of the impact of food and chemical allergies on childhood health. They must also understand that there are no magic bullets. Fortunately, these concepts and their implementation are not difficult. Further, they do not involve any risk to children's health. It is my hope that this book will bring about a greater understanding of the childhood illness-allergy connection and that it will serve as a launching pad for parents, children, and doctors to achieve optimal health and rely less on drugs and surgery.

The Conventional View

Allergy treatments are a multimillion-dollar business with profits that are skyrocketing, thanks to an increasing incidence of allergy-related illnesses. About 130 million school days are missed each year due to hay fever and asthma, and at least one of every six children suffers from an allergy-related health problem. Conventional family doctors, pediatricians, and other specialists usually treat the signs and symptoms of allergy with drugs including antihistamines, decongestants, bronchodilators, and corticosteroids. Desensitization treatments, using weekly allergy injections for several years at a time, are helpful in selected cases, but these are usually given in association with drugs. Diets, vitamins, minerals, and herbs are rarely, if ever, prescribed. Numerous prescription and nonprescription drugs are available to cover up the problem. Unfortunately, although these chemicals are effective in temporarily controlling signs and symptoms, and even lifesaving in rare cases, none of them are curative. Conventional medicine stops short of treating the real causes of allergic disease.

What's Wrong with the Traditional Viewpoint?

The traditional view of the role of allergies in childhood illness has remained unchanged for at least the past two decades. Conventional allergists acknowledge the association between environmental allergies and chronic childhood illnesses such as asthma. The most common environmental allergies treated by traditional allergists, pediatricians, and family doctors are allergies to dust, dust mites, molds, grasses, weeds (e.g., ragweed), and trees.

But chemicals such as formaldehyde, DDT, BHT, MSG, and thousands of other food preservatives, pesticides, herbicides, and disinfectants are not thought by mainstream medical authorities to be responsible for any chronic disease. Some go so far as to say that adverse reactions to common environmental chemicals are not true allergies but a symptom of mental illness. To such allergists, medical conditions such as multiple chemical sensitivity syndrome and twentieth-century disease do not really exist and are the result of a psychiatric problem treatable by antidepressants.

The physical and mental symptoms caused by food and chemical allergies can often leave a child in a general state of misery for years. There is a growing number of environmentally sensitive people, including children, who are dismissed and treated as suffering from psychosomatic illness. The more symptoms patients have, the more likely it is that mainstream doctors will label them as psychiatric cases. The standard dismissal of patients with the phrase "It's all in your head" has forced many victims of allergy to seek help outside of conventional centers.

What Is an Allergy?

I have often wondered why most conventional doctors are so selective in their view of chemicals. Is it not true that they label those who react adversely to chemicals such as antibiotics, analgesics, tranquilizers, and antihistamines as having "an allergy" to those chemicals? Is this just a diagnosis for convenience or a real belief that chemicals can cause allergic reactions?

If you are a parent, you have no doubt heard doctors ask you whether or not your child has an allergy to drugs. If a child who is prescribed the chemical tetracycline—a broad-spectrum antibiotic—suddenly develops bloody diarrhea, generalized edema (swelling caused by abnormal water retention), or hives, he or she is declared to be "allergic to tetracycline." Why is it, then, that if this same child develops a similar reaction to sweeteners, food preservatives, and chemical food dyes, the allergist insists, without objective testing of any kind, that he or she is not allergic to these things? Clearly, there is something very unscientific about the traditional view of allergies. Let's call a spade a spade and define any adverse reaction to a food, chemical, or drug as an allergy.

Mainstream doctors recognize the importance of food allergies in life-threatening conditions such as anaphylactic shock, respiratory arrest, and hives. Peanuts, shellfish, and strawberries are commonly mentioned as the culprits in these situations. The only valid way of diagnosing food allergies, according to traditional medical doctors, is by the skin (scratch) test. If it does not show up on a skin test, it is not an allergy. If a child gets headaches forty-eight hours after consuming dairy products but the skin test is negative, then the headache, even if it occurs every time the child drinks milk, is not caused by an allergy to milk. Conventional doctors refer to these nonallergic food reactions as "food sensitivities." To many wellness- or nutrition-oriented doctors, myself included, this represents a misleading and convenient way of dismissing the serious nature of food allergies. It is certainly not a scientific viewpoint.

A "food sensitivity" is only acknowledged by conventional allergists if an elimination diet (see Chapter 2) confirms its existence. Conventional allergists scoff at the idea that conditions such as migraines, obesity, arthritis, bed-wetting, hyperactivity, learning disabilities, colitis, and a long list of other conditions might be caused by food allergies. Research proves that there is a clear-cut allergy connection.

In fact thousands, if not millions, of children successfully overcome recurrent middle-ear infections, bed-wetting, eczema, asthma, and attention deficit disorder by eliminating certain foods from their diets. The preferred treatments by mainstream doctors for these and dozens of other chronic health disorders continue to be chemicals such as antibiotics, steroid inhalers, cortisone pills and creams, antidepressants, and others. Not only do these drugs have numerous serious side effects such as liver toxicity, yeast infections, bone marrow suppression, constipation, or diarrhea, but they do not get to the source of the problem.

Some people who are more cynical about all this than I am claim that the traditional attitude is spurred on by the profit motive of pharmaceutical and other paramedical concerns. My belief is that the overly conservative traditional view stems more from ignorance due to the lack of instruction given to doctors in medical school on the basics of nutritional medicine and natural therapies.

As you will read later, the prescription-pad drug approach to chronic childhood illnesses is irrational in all but extreme cases. There is a safer and more effective alternative using a combination of self-care and doctor-assisted natural therapies. Improving the quality of the child's diet and lifestyle is very important. Taking food supplements such as vitamins, minerals, amino acids, herbs, and enzymes is also vital. Unfortunately, these approaches alone are often not enough for many children suffering from chronic health problems. Food and chemical allergens must be determined and eliminated from the diet. Additionally, one must take steps to boost the immune system to prevent new allergies from developing.

Food Allergies

One of the first steps in reversing childhood illness is to expand our awareness of food allergy as a prominent cause or aggravating factor in the following conditions:

addiction

anaphylaxis, exercise-induced or otherwise

anxiety

arthritis, including juvenile rheumatoid arthritis

asthma

attention deficit disorder (ADD)

autism

autoimmune diseases (rheumatoid arthritis, lupus, nephritis, nephrotic syndrome, etc.)

bed-wetting (enuresis)

bronchitis

cardiomyopathies

constipation

Crohn's disease

depression

diabetes

diarrhea of unknown cause

dyslexia

eczema

epilepsy and seizure disorders

fatigue, including chronic fatigue syndrome (CFS)

hives (urticaria)

middle-ear infections (otitis media)

migraines

nasal polyps

nightmares

obesity

pain of unknown cause

panic attacks

psoriasis

psychiatric problems of any kind

rashes of unknown cause

recurrent infections of any kind

rhinitis

sinusitis

ulcerative colitis

vascular dysfunctions (e.g., vasculitis)

vitiligo

How do I know if my child has food allergies? Allergies are found in at least sixty percent of all children. The majority of these— especially food allergies—are poorly assessed by conventional skin testing. In fact, the accuracy level of food allergy testing by skin tests is lower than that of flipping a coin to decide whether a food is an allergen (a substance that induces allergic reactions). Skin testing only shows immediate hypersensitivity reactions. Most food allergies occur as delayed reactions showing up a few hours to five days after consumption. For these and other reasons, food allergies can go undetected for years.

Signs and symptoms of food allergy:

Nervous system:

anorexia nervosa, bulimia

anxiety

autism

chronic fatigue

depression

dizziness, faintness

drowsiness, sleepiness after a meal

frequent awakening from sleep

"growing pains"

headaches, migraines

hyperactive behavior

hypoglycemic reactions

inability to return to sleep after awakening

insomnia

memory impairment

muscle aches and pains

panic attacks, rapid heartbeat, irregular or skipped heartbeats

poor school performance

poor work habits

restlessness

schizophrenia

seizures

slurred speech

stuttering

violent, antisocial behavior

Skin, hair, and nails:

abnormal hair loss

brittle and splitting nails

dandruff

dry skin

eczema

itchy scalp

psoriasis

rashes of almost all types

Eyes, ears, nose, and throat:

coated tongue

dark circles under the eyes (allergic shiners)

earaches, recurrent middle-ear infections

excessive mucus production

itchiness at the roof of the mouth

persistent nose-picking

postnasal drip

ringing in the ears (tinnitus)

runny nose

sinusitis

swelling and wrinkles around the eyes

Lungs:

chronic cough of no known cause

congestion

wheezing

Gastrointestinal system:

abdominal cramps or pain

abnormal bowel habits

abnormal food cravings

anal itching

binge eating

bloating, belching, and gas after meals

colic

diarrhea, constipation

mucus and undigested food in the stool

nausea, vomiting

obesity

rapid weight fluctuations

Genitourinary tract:

discharge

recurrent bladder infections

vaginal or scrotal itching

Triggers of food allergies: The most common food allergies are to milk, wheat, citrus products, chocolate, and eggs. These foods are usually eaten on a repetitive, daily basis. One of the many ways in which we can be alerted to a food allergy is through a food craving. Nutritional doctors commonly observe that the foods we crave and eat repeatedly are most likely to be the ones to which we are allergic and physiologically addicted. Food allergy/addiction may be the most common cause of overeating and, hence, obesity.

There are complex biochemical mechanisms that explain the connection between allergy and addiction. One of the best ways to understand the problem is to consider the alcoholic. If one forcibly stops a longtime alcoholic from having alcohol, there are often severe withdrawal reactions. Although the alcohol is damaging to every organ in the person's body, the cravings for this poison are overwhelming. Providing alcohol to such an individual at this time rapidly reverses the withdrawal reactions. In a less dramatic but biochemically similar way, the severely food-addicted child craves the food or combination of foods that causes or aggravates the disease (asthma, arthritis, etc.).

Since an allergic reaction stimulates the increase of adrenaline levels as well as many other biochemical reactions, there is a temporary feeling of wellness or heightened energy whenever one of the "trigger" foods is eaten. Going for long periods of time without the food leads to fatigue until the food is eaten again. So a food allergy develops gradually into an addiction. You can prove this by withholding your child's favorite foods for about a week and then adding them back. If the child is truly allergic to the foods in question, he or she will feel poorly (low energy, headaches, irritability, drowsiness, aggressiveness, etc.) during the period of deprivation. Once the foods are reintroduced, the behavior will shift back temporarily to its opposite.

Environmental Allergies and Chemical Sensitivity

Environmental sensitivity disorders and asthma are increasing at a faster rate for children than for adults. Air pollution and secondhand smoke are responsible for some of this increase, but the role of other environmental toxins must also be acknowledged.

The prevalence of asthma is doubling every twenty years. It increased twenty-nine percent in the United States from 1980 to 1987, from 31.2 per 1,000 to 40.1 per 1,000. While the average increase in asthma diagnoses among U.S. residents of all ages is twenty-nine percent, the increase is forty percent in children, and among females younger than twenty the increase is sixty-nine percent. Asthma also has psychological consequences for children. The U.S. Public Health Service has been quoted as saying, "The importance of emotional factors cannot be ignored; the mental suffering and loss of initiative and confidence that result from repeated asthma attacks can hinder the normal development of children."

High lead levels are reported in up to four million preschoolers. Studies show that children are exposed to higher pesticide levels than adults because their diets contain greater proportions of pesticide-treated produce and that they are not as capable as adults of detoxifying these chemicals. Children are uniquely vulnerable and uniquely affected by environmental toxins, largely because children are physically different from adults in their response to supposedly well-tolerated environmental and food-contaminating chemicals. Foods (milk, dairy products, fruits, vegetables, and grains) purchased at supermarkets and consumed regularly by children are commonly laced with residues of the following pesticides, fungicides, and antiparasitic chemicals:

- benomyl-thiabendazole
- daminozide
- ethylenethiourea (ETU)
- aldicarb
- the organochloride group of pesticides (DDT, DDE, and dieldrin)
- malathione

Exposures to lead, pesticides, secondhand smoke, and other toxic substances is also a contributing factor in middle-ear infections, sudden infant death syndrome, learning disabilities, memory loss, and damage to the central nervous system, the immune system, and the reproductive system. The problem with diagnosing environmental illness is that, in many cases, there are no easily definable symptoms since it can cause all the symptoms of every disease or disorder known to the medical profession. Doctors once used to say that syphilis was the great masquerader because it could mimic the signs and symptoms of any disease. Environmental illness is much the same.

The 60,000 chemicals that are part of a child's everyday life lead to the breakdown of the immune and enzyme systems. Children who suffer from the most severe forms of environmental hypersensitivity have been labeled as having myalgic encephalomyelitis (ME), chronic fatigue syndrome (CFS), or multiple chemical sensitivity (MCS). MCS victims display intense and adverse responses to components of their environment, including water, food, and air. A hypersensitivity to common chemical and environmental stimuli, even at low levels, may trigger reactions that include fatigue, headaches, rashes, difficulty breathing, dizziness, and seizures. Common triggering agents include commonly eaten foods, food additives, antibiotic residues in foods, perfume, scented body sprays, lotions, scented powder, bathroom deodorizers, and many products currently used for cleaning floors, carpets, and other surfaces. The child's body is eventually unable to cope with the chemical overload of the environment, leading to chronic immume impairment and disability.

Despite a growing awareness of its existence, there is still no clear consensus about the status of chemical sensitivity and environmental illness as medical conditions or disabilities. Ongoing research studying the nature of these conditions needs to be conducted in order to define and test for these conditions with a greater degree of accuracy. Although traditional doctors often dismiss diagnoses such as CFS, ME, and MCS as forms of psychiatric problems, MCS is now recognized as a legitimate disability by ten U.S. government agencies as well as numerous state and local governments. MCS sufferers are now protected by the Americans with Disabilities Act. To a less severe extent, children can develop chronic health ailments as a result of food and chemical allergies that still allow them to go to school and function at an acceptable, albeit impaired, level with conditions such as allergic rhinitis, asthma, learning disabilities, and ADD.

Human breast milk is contaminated with more than one hundred industrial chemicals, including pesticides. This is not meant to say that women should not breast-feed their infants because, relatively speaking, breast-fed infants have far healthier immune systems than bottle-fed infants.

Multiple Chemical Sensitivity Syndrome

Multiple chemical sensitivity syndrome is defined by specialists of environmental medicine as an abnormal response of the body to everyday substances such as food, chemicals, drugs, air pollution, perfumes, pollens, dust, and molds. The severe reactions can be debilitating, affecting the eyes, ears, skin, nose, throat, lungs, stomach, muscles, joints, nervous system, brain, and urinary tract. This environmental hypersensitivity syndrome is thought to be the result of a combination of factors that include heredity, acute chemical exposure, intense life stresses, poor nutritional status, and viral, bacterial, or fungal infections.

Common symptoms of environmental hypersensitivity are headaches, asthma, nasal congestion, nausea, bloating, joint pain, muscle pain and weakness, fatigue, sleepiness, anxiety, poor concentration, confusion, depression, mood swings, puffy eyes, and weight loss. Many familiar illnesses are the result of reactions to a variety of substances found in the home or school. Increasing numbers of children suffering from disorders such as sleep disturbances, learning disabilities, hyperactivity, diabetes, and inflammations of the blood vessels, colon, and bladder, as well as a host of other inflammatory diseases including rheumatoid arthritis, can be directly related to environmental hypersensitivity. The reactions are usually to synthetic toxic chemicals increasingly found in what we eat, drink, breathe, wear, or touch that cannot be entirely eliminated from our day-to-day environments.

Air, water, and food are contaminated with at least 100,000 chemicals in commercial use today. There are thousands of new chemicals added to the environment yearly, with the long-term toxic effects being unknown. Some of these chemicals include derivatives or compounds containing chlorine, fluorine, lead, mercury, cadmium, aluminum, pesticides, herbicides, insecticides, chemical fertilizers, ozone, formaldehyde, phenols, solvents, pentachlorophenols, PCBs, asbestos, sulfur dioxide, and derivatives of gas, oil, and coal. It is estimated that the average North American child consumes eight to fifteen pounds of harmful chemicals each year. About five pounds of this are stored in body fat or deep muscle tissues.

Psychological stress caused by family problems, alcoholism, the death of a parent, and poverty can certainly weaken the immune system of any child. But to think that chemical, physical, and biological poisons have nothing to do with immune system damage and allergies is a form of denial. To say that people who have developed sensitivities and chronic illnesses are simply suffering from a psychiatric problem is to add insult to injury. Although it is true that emotional stress is often responsible for the appearance of many suboptimal health conditions, the chemical stressors in our environment cannot easily be explained away by labeling severely allergic people as having some form of depression worthy only of psychiatric intervention. Yet this is exactly what often happens to the chemically hypersensitive, who are able to tolerate only a limited variety of foods, locations, and climates.

Digestion and Allergies

The front line of the immune system's defenses against allergens and toxins is the digestive system. If there is already an impairment of the digestive system, food and chemical allergies are more likely to develop. Conversely, an inherited or acquired food or chemical allergy can create an eventual impairment in the gastrointestinal tract. In that sense, digestive problems can both cause and be the result of food and chemical allergies. Chronic digestive problems result in malnutrition and immune system impairment. This happens because essential nutrients may be malabsorbed, and a damaged gastrointestinal tract can allow the bloodstream to be bombarded with incompletely digested foods and unwanted bacteria, fungi, and parasites and their toxins. Food allergies may cause the gut injury, and gut injury can cause reactions that look like food allergies. Additionally, partially digested and undigested foods enter the large intestine or colon where the bowel flora can become imbalanced in favor of candida, putrefactive bacteria, and parasites. The toxins produced can lead to inflammation, diarrhea, constipation, diverticulosis(the development of tiny projections of tissue from the gastrointestinal tract), diverticulitis, appendicitis, or colitis.

The often-used expression "You are what you eat" is only partially correct. It is more accurate to say, "You are what you absorb." One can have a most perfect diet, take vitamin and mineral tablets, and still be very ill if one's digestion is poor. Absorption of essential nutrients into the bloodstream could then be faulty and lead to numerous vitamin and mineral deficiencies. This, in turn, can weaken the immune system's ability to deal with invading organisms such as bacteria, fungi, and parasites. One sign of poor assimilation is the finding of completely undigested vitamin or mineral tablets in the toilet bowl after a bowel movement. This is a common sign in children with multiple food allergies.

If digestive function is impaired, partially digested protein molecules can enter the bloodstream and elicit an immune response. If this immune response occurs in the respiratory tract, the end result could be asthma, bronchitis, sinusitis, or a middle-ear infection. If it happens in the joints, it can trigger rheumatoid arthritis flare-ups. If immune reactions take place in the nervous system, the end result might very well be attention deficit disorder or depression. The genetic weakness of the individual is likely to determine the site of inflammation and eventual disease.

The Role of Stomach Acidity

It has been demonstrated by researchers that asthmatic children can decrease the severity and frequency of attacks simply by taking a supplement that increases the acidity of the stomach. Supplements such as glutamic acid, betaine and pepsin hydrochloride, bromelain, apple cider vinegar, lemon juice, and stomach bitters can all help improve the breakdown of protein and prevent the absorption of undigested polypeptides (protein molecules) that cause an immune response leading to a asthmatic attack. Low or nonexistent stomach acidity—hypochlorhydria—is a common finding not only in asthma but in many other diseases of the immune system.

Stomach acid is absolutely essential for digesting protein and for the absorption of vitamins and trace minerals such as iron, copper, manganese, and dozens of others. Since it has been estimated that about half the population of North America has low stomach acidity, it should not be surprising that a long list of maladies is associated with low or absent stomach acidity.

Conditions associated with stomach acid deficiency:

acne

anemia of many kinds (iron, copper, vitamin B-12)

asthma

autoimmune diseases (rheumatoid arthritis, lupus, vitiligo, multiple sclerosis, scleroderma)

candida syndrome

colitis

digestive symptoms of unknown cause (gas, bloating, nausea, diarrhea, constipation, belching, heartburn, cramping, smelly stools)

food allergies

irritable bowel syndrome

parasites

vitamin and mineral deficiencies (B-12, iron, copper, zinc, manganese, calcium)

The combination of stomach acid deficiency and food allergies can perpetuate a vicious cycle. Low hydrochloric acid levels in the stomach can worsen food reactions or allergies. Eating allergenic foods repeatedly can cause damage to the lining of the stomach, leading to low or nonexistent production of hydrochloric acid by the parietal cells (stomach cells responsible for acid production). This is particularly true with those who are heavy consumers of milk and other dairy products.

Antacids and acid-suppressing drugs such as cimetidine and ranitidine can lead to infections because they eliminate the protective effect of hydrochloric acid. But one must be careful with acid supplementation because excess acid can cause severe heartburn and possibly lead to gastric irritation and bleeding.

The need for acid supplementation should be determined by tests ordered by a natural health care practitioner. These tests include the CDSA (comprehensive digestive and stool analysis) and a direct stomach acid determination with special pH-measuring instruments. Live-cell microscopic examination (dark-field microscopy) is another test worth doing since it can provide indirect evidence of low hydrochloric acid levels.

The Role of Digestive Enzymes

Some children not only have a weakness in stomach acid but are also deficient in pancreatic and intestinal digestive enzymes, which are needed for the breakdown of proteins and carbohydrates. Pancreatic digestive enzymes (amylase, protease, lipase, trypsin, and others) normally form a line of protection that helps prevent infections from pathogenic bacteria, fungi, and parasites that enter the body through the gastrointestinal tract. The level of pancreatic digestive juice is often low in children with digestive problems and many other diseases associated with food allergies.

Undigested vegetables found in the stool and poor tolerance to high-complex-carbohydrate foods (starches, high-fiber cereal grains, legumes) are often signs of weak pancreatic enzyme production. In such cases, the best treatment is to both eliminate the allergenic foods from the diet and supplement the diet with either pancreatic digestive enzymes or plant-based intestinal enzymes. An extreme form of this problem occurs in cystic fibrosis, where there is a complete lack of pancreatic digestive enzymes. Unfortunately, many milder forms of this condition are passed off as a psychiatric problem. Symptoms that might tip you off that your child is suffering from low pancreatic digestive enzymes include constipation, excessive belching, gas, cramps, flatulence, or foul, smelly stools.

It should be noted here that many natural health care practitioners find that the plant-source digestive enzymes work somewhat better than the animal-source variety derived from beef, pork, or lamb. The reason for this is that animal-based enzymes can only work well at a high pH (alkaline) level. The pH in the intestine is alkaline, while that of the stomach is much more acid. Animal-based enzymes do not work in the low-pH, highly acid stomach. Plant-based enzymes, on the other hand, work well in both acid and alkaline environments. Plant enzymes are similar to pancreatic and intestinal digestive enzymes except that they are derived from fungi. Examples of plant-based enzymes include bromelain and papain, two common health-food-store remedies. Bromelain is a proteolytic (protein-digesting) enzyme found in pineapples that not only helps improve digestion but has been found to be effective in obesity and many inflammatory conditions such as tendonitis, bursitis, and plantar fascitis. Papain is a weaker proteolytic enzyme derived from papaya.

The Leaky Gut

Understanding the leaky gut phenomenon not only helps us see why allergies and autoimmune diseases develop, but also helps us with safe and effective therapies to bring the body back into balance. An autoimmune disease is defined as one in which the immune system makes antibodies against its own tissues. Common childhood autoimmune diseases in this category include alopecia areata, juvenile rheumatoid arthritis, fibromyalgia, chronic fatigue syndrome, vitiligo, urticaria (hives), and juvenile diabetes. Physicians are increasingly recognizing the importance of the gastrointestinal tract in the development of allergic or autoimmune disease.

The leaky gut syndrome is a very common problem and rapidly increasing, especially in children suffering from recurrent infections of any kind who are constantly on antibiotics. Leaky gut syndrome is at least as common as all the immune system diseases put together. The basic defect in leaky gut syndrome is an intestinal lining that is more permeable than normal. This means that large spaces are present between the cells of the gut wall, allowing the entrance of bacteria, fungi, parasites, toxins, undigested protein, fat, and waste material into the bloodstream. The gut becomes leaky in the sense that substances (undigested proteins, toxins, etc.) normally not absorbed in the healthy state pass through a damaged, hyperpermeable, porous, or "leaky" gut. This can be verified by special gut-permeability urine tests or by microscopic examination of the lining of the intestinal wall and the bloodstream using phase-contrast microscopy (also known as dark-field microscopy).

The leaky gut syndrome is caused by inflammation of the gut lining (see the list on page 24 for causes of the inflammation). Inflammation causes the spaces between the cells to enlarge, allowing the absorption of large protein molecules which are usually broken down to much smaller pieces before being absorbed through the normally small spaces between the gut-lining cells. The immune system then makes antibodies against these large molecules because it recognizes them as a foreign, invading substance. Since a healthy gut would not allow the presence of such large proteins in the bloodstream, the immune system starts treating them as if they had to be destroyed. Antibodies are made against the proteins and the previously harmless foods.

These antibodies can then get into various tissues and trigger an inflammatory reaction when their corresponding food is consumed. This occurs because body tissues have antigenic sites (locations on cells seen as similar to invading substances) very similar to those on the foods, bacteria, parasites, candida, or fungi. Autoantibodies are thus created, and inflammation becomes chronic. If this inflammation occurs in a joint, autoimmune arthritis (childhood rheumatoid arthritis) develops. If it occurs in the brain, seizures or epilepsy may be the result. If it occurs in the blood vessels, vasculitis (inflammation of the blood vessels) is the resulting autoimmune problem. If the antibodies end up attacking the lining of the gut itself, the result may be colitis or Crohn's disease. If it occurs in the lungs, asthma is triggered on a delayed basis every time the individual consumes the food which stimulated the production of the antibodies in the first place.

It is easy to see that practically any organ or body tissue can become affected by food allergies created by the leaky gut. Symptoms, especially those seen in conditions such as chronic fatigue syndrome, can be multiple and severely debilitating.

The inflammation that causes the leaky gut syndrome also damages the protective coating of antibodies of the IgA family (a family of antibodies produced by the immune system to protect the body from invading microbes) normally present in a healthy gut. Since IgA helps us ward off infections, with leaky gut problems we become less resistant to viruses, bacteria, parasites, and candida. These microbes are then able to invade the bloodstream and colonize almost any body tissue or organ. When this occurs in the gums, periodontal disease results. If it happens in the jaw, tooth extraction or root canals might be necessary to cure the infection.

In addition to the creation of food allergies, a leaky gut allows the bloodstream to be invaded by bacteria, fungi, and parasites that, in the healthy state, would not penetrate the protective barrier of the gut. These microbes and their toxins, if present in large enough amounts, can overwhelm the liver's detoxification capacity. This can result in symptoms such as confusion, memory loss, brain fog, or facial swelling when the individual is exposed to an inhalant (e.g., perfume or cigarette smoke) to which he or she had no adverse reactions prior to developing leaky gut syndrome.

Leaky gut syndrome also causes a long list of mineral deficiencies because the inflammation process damages the carrier proteins in the gastrointestinal tract that are needed to transport minerals from the intestine to the blood. For example, magnesium deficiency is a common finding in conditions such as fibromyalgia, despite a high magnesium intake through the diet and supplementation. If the carrier protein for magnesium is damaged, magnesium deficiency develops as a result of malabsorption. Muscle pain and spasms can occur as a result. Similarly, zinc deficiency due to malabsorption can result in hair loss or baldness, as occurs in alopecia areata. Copper deficiency can occur in an identical way, leading to high blood cholesterol levels and joint pain. Further, bone problems develop as a result of the malabsorption of calcium, boron, silicon, and manganese.

Causes of inflammation leading to the leaky gut syndrome:

• Antibiotics, because they cause abnormal flora in the gastro-intestinal tract (bacteria, parasites, candida, fungi)

• Caffeine (strong gut irritant found in chocolate and cola beverages)

• Chemicals (dyes, preservatives, peroxidized fats) in fermented and processed food such as vinegar and cheeses

• Enzyme deficiencies (e.g., celiac disease, lactase deficiency causing lactose intolerance)

• Foods and beverages, which are contaminated by bacteria like *helicobacter pylori, klebsiella, citrobacter, pseudomonas* and others such as beef, pork, poultry, and seafood.

• Foods and beverages such as tap water, fruits, and vegetables which are contaminated by parasites like *giardia lamblia, cryptosporidium, blastocystis hominis,* and others

• High refined carbohydrate diet (e.g., candy bars, cookies, cake, soft drinks, white bread)

• Mold and fungal mycotoxins in stored grains, fruit, and refined carbohydrates

• NSAIDs (nonsteroidal anti-inflammatory drugs) such as ibuprofen, indomethacin, etc.

• Prescription corticosteroids (e.g., prednisone)

• Prescription hormones such as the birth control pill (often prescribed by gynecologists even for young girls with menstrual problems)

Leaky gut patients can help themselves by chewing their food more thoroughly, following the basic rules of food-combining, eating frequent small meals rather than three large ones, and taking more time with their meals. Proper food combining means to eat high-protein foods like meat separately from high-carbohydrate foods such as potatoes. In other words, do not eat foods like meats, fish, poultry, eggs, and dairy products in the same meal as starches like breads, crackers, pasta, cereals, or potatoes. Always eat raw fruit alone or about half an hour before a meal to prevent maldigestion. Cooked fruit is okay to eat during or after a meal.

Gastrointestinal function can be improved with a juice fast or a hypoallergenic, higher-fiber diet and supplements such as *lactobacillus acidophilus* and *bifidus*, as well as FOSs (fructooligosaccharides) derived from Jerusalem artichoke, chicory, the dahlia plant, or burdock root.

Supplements beneficial in the treatment of leaky gut syndrome:

• Amino acids: L-glutamine, N-acetyl-glucosamine (NAG)

• Antioxidants: carotenoids, B complex, vitamin C, vitamin E, zinc, selenium, germanium, coenzyme Q10, and bioflavonoids, especially quercetin, catechin, hesperidin, rutin, and proanthocyanidins (pycnogenols, grape-seed extract, pine-bark extract, bilberry)

- Combination green foods which contain spirulina, chlorella, or blue-green algae, wheat grass, green barley, green kamut, and alfalfa

- Essential fatty acids (EFAs): milled flax, flaxseed oil, evening primrose oil, borage oil, olive oil, fish oils, black currant seed oil

- Herbs and plant extracts: various high-chlorophyll green drinks such as spirulina, chlorella, and blue-green algae; kudzu, burdock, slippery elm, Turkish rhubarb, sheep sorrel, licorice root, ginger root, goldenseal, bismuth, and bentonite

- Natural digestive enzymes: from plants (e.g., bromelain, papain) or pancreatic animal tissues (porcine, bovine, lamb) and aloe vera juice with a high MPS (mucopolysaccharides) concentration

- Soluble fiber: psyllium seed husks and powder, apple or citrus pectin, rice-derived gamma oryzanol

- Stomach-acidity-enhancing supplements: betaine and pepsin, glutamic acid, stomach bitters, apple cider vinegar

Because of the increasing recognition of chronic fatigue syndrome, the leaky gut syndrome, and multiple chemical sensitivity, a number of supplement companies have been marketing powdered formulations suitable for children aged four to twelve that contain most of the nutrients mentioned above in one convenient package.

Additional Challenges to a Child's Immune System

A large number of physical factors must be added to the list of assaults on children's immune systems. These are the extremes of heat, cold, weather cycles, noise, positive and negative ions, electromagnetic radiation, and radioactivity from X-rays, food irradiation, and radon gas. In addition, biological stressors include antibiotic-resistant bacteria, viruses, molds, candida, parasites, irradiated foods, animal dander, dust, and pollens from trees, grasses, and weeds.

Drug-Resistant Parasites

> Parasites are the missing diagnosis in the genesis of many chronic health problems, including diseases of the gastrointestinal tract and endocrine system.
>
> —*Hermann R. Bueno, M.D.*

Amoebae, worms, and other parasites are increasingly being seen in children. Some secrete toxins as part of their elimination process. Those toxins are capable of eliciting a strong immune system reaction like hives, wheezing, gastrointestinal distress, and other allergy-like symptoms.

Parasites are often difficult to eradicate, and treatment might last a year or longer for complete clearing. The incidence of parasitic diseases in North America is skyrocketing because of increased international travel, contamination of the water and food supply, and the overuse of chemicals, mercury, and prescription antibiotics. These organisms can be microscopic in size or visible to the naked eye as wormlike creatures such as pinworms. Tapeworms, hookworms, and a long list of amoebae are far more common in the North American population than conventional medical experts have led the population to believe. In fact, according to Anne Louise Gittleman, author of the book *Guess What Came to Dinner,* parasites are present in eight out of every ten individuals. Filarial worms, hookworms, whipworms, pinworms, and flatworms affect more than two billion people around the world, causing a long list of afflictions ranging from elephantiasis to blindness to serious intestinal problems.

Most specialists in parasitology say that at least forty percent of the world's population is infected by worms. It matters not whether one is wealthy or poor. Parasites attack all socioeconomic groups, including famous movie stars and the families of reputable cardiac surgeons. The highest concentrations of parasites are found in commercial pork products (bacon, ham, hot dogs, cold cuts, pork chops, etc.). Beef, chicken, lamb, and even fish can also be contaminated. Sushi from many parts of the world contains the larvae of several species of parasitic worms. Cows fed the dried dead flesh of other cows often have parasites of many kinds embedded in their organs. Microwaving and high temperature are usually ineffective at eradicating these ubiquitous organisms. So is chlorinated tap water. Small wonder that vegetarian eating has gained in popularity.

The worst outbreak of a waterborne disease in modern U.S. history occurred in Milwaukee, Wisconsin, in 1993. Severe bouts of watery diarrhea struck an estimated 403,000 people, and over 100 people are estimated to have died from the *cryptosporidium* parasite. The same parasite was present in three watersheds of the Greater Vancouver, B.C. regional district's water system, according to its 1991 annual report. The Greater Vancouver regional district uses chlorination for water treatment, but *cryptosporidium* is highly resistant to chlorine.

Although it is known that the use of ozone is an effective way of eliminating *cryptosporidium* from drinking water, there is a great deal of resistance to converting the chlorination process to ozonation. Another alternative to chlorination is using a filter no larger than 1 mm in diameter. Anything larger will allow small parasites like *cryptosporidium* to get into the drinking water.

Chlorination of the water supply is not enough protection against the majority of parasites. Epidemic outbreaks of parasites such as *giardia, cryptosporidium,* and *endolimax nana* in cities using chlorination are clear evidence that something more than chlorine is required to eradicate parasites from the food supply. Nearly one hundred percent of European cities use ozonation to purify drinking water.

Signs of parasites in the human body:
- bed-wetting
- blurry or unclear vision (especially when bending over or standing up)

- burning sensation in the stomach
- chest pain
- damp lips at night, dry lips during the day
- drooling while asleep
- eating more than normal but still feeling hungry
- fast heartbeat
- gas and bloating
- grinding teeth while asleep
- itchy rectum, nose, and ears
- loss of desire for food
- numb hands
- pain in the back, thighs, and shoulders
- pain in the navel
- unclear thinking, forgetfulness, lethargy, slow reflexes
- yellowish face

Even if children do not have any of these symptoms, naturopaths often recommend doing a parasite cleanse at least twice
a year for prevention. A parasite cleanse involves using some of
the natural remedies listed later. The reason a parasite cleanse is
suggested is that stool analysis does not always reveal the parasite. Certainly, in the allergic child, a parasite cleanse can make
all the difference in the reversal of chronic illness.

The most accurate way of making a diagnosis of parasites is
by what is known as a purged stool sample. This is one in which a
complete evacuation of gastrointestinal contents is achieved
through the use of a saline (salt solution) laxative. Random stool
analysis (not purged) will miss the diagnosis in over fifty percent
of the cases. Many labs in the United States and Canada do not
examine even purged stools with the appropriate stains or
equipment. Most natural health care practitioners, as well as a
growing number of conventional doctors, recommend using
Great Smokies Diagnostic Lab (see reference section) and

others like it that specialize in detailed stool analysis. Dark-field microscopy is another way in which the parasite problem might be diagnosed, although this is controversial at the time of this writing. Any informed medical doctor, naturopath, osteopath, or nutritionally trained chiropractor can make the diagnosis and initiate therapy.

A safe and effective therapy against parasites is the use of digestive supplements. Some acid and digestive enzyme supplements one could consider with monitoring by a natural health care practitioner include:

- Aloe vera juice
- Apple cider vinegar
- Bromelain
- Glutamic acid hydrochloride
- Kombucha herb tea—this product also supplies the gastro-intestinal tract with many beneficial bacteria, amino acids, B vitamins, and enzymes
- Pepsin hydrochloride
- Swedish Bitters

Aside from prescription drugs, the following is a list of nat-ural antiparasitic herbs that are often as effective as or superior to more conventional treatments:

- Apple pectin powder
- Bismuth, slippery elm, goldenseal, and bentonite
- Black walnut, green hulls, black seed cloves, southern wood, bitter sophora, wormwood, peppermint leaves, grapefruit seed extract
- Garlic (allicin-containing health food store brands)
- Milled flaxseed, psyllium seed powder
- Olive oil

Drinking Water

You will observe with great concern how long a useful truth may be known to exist before it is generally known and practiced.

—*Benjamin Franklin*

Dangers of fluoridated water: Fluoride can deactivate many enzymes in a child's body which might provide protection against possible allergens. In small amounts, fluoride might be tolerated. Unfortunately, this is not the case in North America, where children are being overexposed to this mineral.

Fluoridation has never been governed by science. The U.S. Food and Drug Administration (FDA) has no proof of fluoride safety or effectiveness. The FDA has no drug application on record for fluoride, and none has ever been submitted. The National Institute of Dental Research (NIDR) has no proof of fluoride safety or effectiveness. The American Academy of Pediatric Dentistry has no proof of fluoride safety or effectiveness. Nearly one hundred percent of all western European countries refuse to use fluoridation because of the many health concerns.

The case against fluoride:

1. Fluoride is deposited in bone and soft tissues, where it has the potential to cause serious harm, such as brittle bones and cancer, in later years.

2. Fluoride causes a condition known as fluorosis, which can best be described as opaque white spots on the teeth and brown, ugly teeth. Fluorosis currently affects one out of five or more children in the United States, although it is rarely seen in California (possibly because California is the least fluoridated state, with less than sixteen percent of the population drinking artificially fluoridated water). Dental fluorosis is not just a cosmetic problem, as many dentists and the public health services claim it to be. It is a visible sign of fluoride poisoning and an indication of permanent damage to the teeth.

3. Fluoride is ineffective in reducing tooth decay. Several well-conducted studies show no correlation between the level of fluoride in water and cavities. Tooth decay is more highly correlated to the educational and economic level of the parents.

4. Fluoride is an equivocal carcinogen—one that is not universally accepted as a cause of cancer—according to the National Cancer Institute Toxicological Program.

5. The FDA considers fluoride an unapproved new drug with no proof of safety or effectiveness. It also does not consider fluoride an essential nutrient.

6. The International Academy of Oral Medicine and Toxicology has classified fluoride as an unapproved dental treatment due to its high toxicity.

The original studies by H. Trendly Dean on fluoridation, which led to the decision to allow fluoridation of municipal water supplies, were unscientific by the author's own criteria. The studies did not look at other minerals in the water and their interactions. They also did not take into account the differences between "natural fluoride" (CaF) and fluoride waste products (NaF)—the harmful combination of fluoride with other minerals or chemical compounds in water. The study had little or no statistical analysis and only reported a portion of the data gathered while ignoring important data that cast a bad light on fluoridation.

Chlorinated tap water: Chlorine is a greenish yellow, poisonous, gaseous chemical element with a disagreeable odor, used in bleaching agents, water purification, and various industrial processes and as a lung irritant in chemical warfare. Chlorine has been documented to aggravate asthma, especially in children who make frequent use of chlorinated swimming pools.

Chlorine attacks bacteria in drinking water, but in the process of disinfecting, new chemical compounds of chlorine are created. Chlorine molecules react with otherwise harmless organic material present in the raw water supply, creating a group of chlorinated chemical compounds called trihalomethanes

(THMs). THMs are tasteless and odorless, but they are considered human carcinogens. They also depress the central nervous system and can cause damage to the liver and kidneys. These chemicals, also known as organochlorides, do not degrade well and are generally stored in the fatty tissues of the body. Organochlorides can suppress immune system function, interfere with the natural controls of cell growth, and cause mutations by altering DNA.

Chlorinated tap water is a skin irritant and can be associated with many types of rashes, including eczema. Chlorinated water can destroy polyunsaturated fatty acids and vitamin E and generate toxins capable of causing free radical damage or oxidation (see Chapter 6 for a more detailed discussion of oxidation, free radical damage, and antioxidants). This might explain why supplementation of the diet with essential fatty acids such as flaxseed oil, evening primrose oil, borage oil, and antioxidants (vitamin E, selenium, and others) helps so many cases of eczema.

Chlorinated water destroys many of the intestinal flora that help in the digestion of food and protect the body from harmful pathogens. It is not uncommon for chronic digestive disorders as well as chronic skin conditions such as acne, psoriasis, seborrhea, and eczema to clear up or be significantly improved by switching to unchlorinated drinking water and supplementing the diet with *lactobacillus acidophilus* and *bifidus*.

Drinking water recommendations: Bottled spring water is the best drinking water, but the source should be a real spring and not filtered tap water. When it comes to commercially sold water, false advertisers are everywhere. It is a good idea to call various consumer agencies and check the source of the water you and your children drink. Water should be regularly tested for contaminants. You have every right to ask for the testing schedule and the list of what a company tests for. Look for water that has not been "improved" by the addition of chlorine, magnesium, or softeners. Water should be bottled in glass, not plastic, containers; plastic tends to combine with water, creating toxic compounds.

Safe, clean, bottled spring water is either unavailable or unaffordable to many people. Reverse osmosis and distillation are the best alternatives to spring water; they are the only way to reliably remove the fluoride and chlorine from tap water. Carbon filters can become contaminated with bacteria and must be replaced often. Distilled and reverse-osmosis water are devoid of minerals, so if you use them, you should take supplemental colloidal minerals daily.

In the absence of reverse-osmosis filtering devices or distillation, you can evaporate ninety percent or more of the chlorine and fluoride and its by-products from tap water by putting the water in a blender for fifteen minutes with the lid off. If you don't have a blender, mix your water in a bowl with a spoon. Be sure to do this in a well-ventilated room to minimize damage from inhaling the released chlorine gases.

You should check any beverages that you purchase and ingest on a regular basis for the source of the water to see if it is fluoridated. If it says "filtered water" on the ingredients label, this does not necessarily mean that the water is nonfluoridated, unless a reverse-osmosis filter was used.

Avoid fluoridated toothpastes, and purchase sweetener-free, fluoride-free toothpaste at a health food store. Sweeteners and other chemicals in toothpastes stimulate the growth of unfriendly microbes such as candida, bacteria, and parasites. Make sure the toothpaste you use has no saccharine, sodium lauryl sulfate, or other unhealthy chemicals. Use baking soda or tea tree oil and water if you can't find an appropriate toothpaste.

Mercury Amalgam

If everyone is thinking alike, no one is thinking.

—*Benjamin Franklin*

Most parents never give a second thought to the safety of mercury dental amalgams placed in the teeth of their children. Mercury, however, is capable of eliciting negative immune system reactions as well as neurological abnormalities. As such, mercury may be responsible for exaggerated immune system reactions in children such as asthma, hives, chronic fatigue syndrome, and seizure disorders.

Mercury contained in dental restorations is hazardous to the human body. Amalgams are mixtures of metals used to fill the teeth; mercury amalgam contains fifty percent mercury along with silver, tin, copper, and sometimes zinc, indium, palladium, or small amounts of cadmium.

Conventional dental authorities in North America and Britain are attempting to defuse the mercury amalgam toxicity issue by ignoring the existence of voluminous amounts of scientific research. Despite the fact that over one hundred published scientific papers directly implicate mercury released from amalgam restorations as a major contributing factor in chronic illness, groups such as the American Dental Association (ADA) and the Canadian Dental Association (CDA) refuse to acknowledge their existence.

Persistent denial of the dangers of mercury in dental fillings comes in the form of written pronouncements and angry attacks in the media by ivory-tower heads of dental associations. The American Dental Association (ADA) has even published literature stating that any dentist who removes amalgam restorations due to mercury toxicity is to be considered unethical.

The American Academy of Head, Neck, and Facial Pain has decided to take a stand against the ADA and its outdated policy on mercury dental fillings. In recent literature, this group states:

> We feel the evidence is too overwhelming to continue to practice in ignorance and avoidance of the facts. The Board of Directors, under the name of our Academy, has written a petition to several agencies (the FDA, OSHA, NIH, NIDR, U.S. Public Health Service, and the National Institute of Environmental Health Services) asking that all past and current scientific literature concerning mercury and dental amalgams be re-evaluated.

What is the evidence incriminating the mercury dental filling? The following are documented facts about mercury amalgam toxicity taken from the scientific literature:

1. Mercury damages DNA, alters the structure of proteins, disrupts the communication between cells, induces free radical tissue damage, and inhibits antioxidant enzymes such as glutathione peroxidase. Mercury from a single dental filling is enough to inhibit the activity of white blood cells. Mercury can indirectly increase antibiotic-resistant oral and intestinal bacteria, impair kidney function, and induce autoimmune diseases such as multiple sclerosis, systemic lupus erythematosus, and chronic fatigue syndrome.

   Eight of the eleven symptom criteria set for chronic fatigue syndrome by the Centers for Disease Control are well-known symptoms of mercury poisoning. The World Health Organization (WHO) has recently stated that "it is not scientifically possible to set a level for mercury in blood or urine below which mercury-related symptoms will not occur."

   The medical literature reports a long list of signs and symptoms alleviated by replacement of mercury dental fillings including allergies, gastrointestinal problems of all types, tension headaches, migraine headaches, unexplained hair loss in women, eczema, asthma, multiple sclerosis, lupus, Parkinson's disease, and urinary tract problems.

2. Mercury is continually released in the mouth from amalgam restorations. Those with amalgam fillings have an average mercury vapor concentration ten times higher than in people without such fillings. Chewing gum, brushing teeth, and drinking hot beverages all increase mercury release.

3. Mercury vapors from dental amalgams are absorbed directly into the blood and almost all body tissues including the oral cavity, the lungs, and the gastrointestinal tract. Mercury fillings in pregnant women also affect the growing fetus. Autopsies done on aborted human babies found that mercury levels in the brain, liver, and kidney correlated significantly with the number of amalgam fillings in their mothers.

4. Mercury levels in the blood, urine, brain, nerves, endocrine glands, and kidneys increase in direct proportion to the num-

ber of amalgam restorations present in the mouth. Studies indicate that eighty percent of inhaled mercury vapor is absorbed into the bloodstream. There is a direct transport of mercury through the peripheral nerves and into the central nervous system. Autopsy studies reveal statistically significant correlations between measured mercury tissue concentrations and the number of amalgam fillings.

5. Based on extensive scientific documentation, several world governments (e.g., Germany, Austria, Sweden, Norway) have either banned the use of mercury dental amalgams outright or severely curtailed their use, especially in pregnant women or those with kidney problems.

It must be stressed that the removal and replacement of amalgam fillings releases mercury vapors and can worsen symptoms, especially in highly sensitive individuals such as those suffering from chronic fatigue syndrome or severe environmental hypersensitivity syndromes. Some individuals should therefore not consider replacing mercury fillings at all or only very carefully on the advice of their natural health care practitioner or medical specialist.

To prevent or offset mercury damage from the replacement of dental amalgams, one can follow a high-fiber diet, eat more garlic and onions, drink distilled water, and supplement with high doses of beta carotene, vitamin A, vitamin C, selenium, vitamin E, aloe vera juice, green drinks such as barley green, chlorella, spirulina, and blue-green algae, and high-sulfur-content amino acids such as cysteine, methionine, N-acetyl-cysteine, and glutathione. This regimen will lessen the effects of amalgam fillings even if they aren't replaced and is also acceptable as a way of preventing free radical damage to the body by any toxic heavy metal. To find a dentist in your area who knows about mercury alternatives, contact the Consumer Health Organization of Canada, DAMS (Dental Amalgam Mercury Syndrome), or the Environmental Dental Association (see Appendix IV).

Sugar

Sugar hinders the body's immune system and predisposes children to infections and allergies. The shape, activity, and number of white blood cells are adversely affected by heavy sugar consumption. Sugar is the single most underrated cause of immune system impairment. Flu and other respiratory tract or middle-ear infections can often be traced to heavy sugar consumption after holidays (Halloween, Christmas), when a lot of sweets are consumed.

Sugar goes by many names, including sucrose, fructose, brown sugar, invert sugar, dextrose, maltose, lactose, xylitol, sorbitol, honey, and molasses. White flour products (white breads, cakes, pastries, cookies, pasta, pancakes, donuts, etc.) are not sugar in themselves but are quickly converted in the body to simple sugars; one slice of white bread is equivalent to one teaspoon of sugar.

Sugar is hidden in many commercially available foods. For example, a tablespoon of ketchup contains one teaspoon of sugar. Some soft drinks contain up to twelve teaspoons of sugar per eight ounces. Jelly beans and marshmallows derive one hundred percent of their calories from sugar. Even some unsweetened fruit juices contain the equivalent of ten teaspoons of sugar and should be avoided by diabetics, hypoglycemics, and those with high blood levels of triglycerides. Mayonnaise, cereals, breads, mustard, relish, peanut butter, gravies, sauces, TV dinners, and even drugs are hidden sources of large amounts of sugar.

Sugar and sugar equivalents, such as white bread, cause a rapid rise in blood glucose and insulin levels shortly after ingestion. The more sugar that is consumed, the more insulin must be made by the pancreas. Eventually the pancreas gets overworked. If sugar intake remains excessive and frequent, blood glucose levels crash below acceptable levels, producing transient low blood sugar attacks (hypoglycemia). These may be experienced as anxiety, panic, headaches, sudden fatigue, sleepiness after eating, mood swings, behavior disorders, hyperactivity, and a craving for more sweets. The adrenal glands—the body's anti-stress glands—in turn get overstressed, leading to chronic tiredness and poor school performance.

Other terms used to describe the symptoms of nutritional stress caused by sugar are "idiopathic post-prandial syndrome," "nutritionally induced chronic endocrinopathy" (NICE), and "adrenal insufficiency." One endocrine gland after the other may become involved (thyroid, pituitary, ovaries, etc.). Full-blown diseases such as diabetes, hypothyroidism, and Addison's disease result after years of unabated nutritional stress created by a high sugar intake.

Many consumers are aware of the dangers of high sugar consumption and have therefore opted for other sweeteners, both artificial and natural, in ever-growing numbers. Are any of these better or worse than sugar, and why?

Sugar alternatives—natural sweeteners:

- Sucanat (granulated cane juice) is whole-cane sugar, calories and all, with the water removed. This is only slightly healthier than table sugar (sucrose) because of its low content of vitamins and minerals. Sucanat in small amounts is appropriate in the diets of healthy children and adults, but it is still to be avoided by diabetics, hypoglycemics, and children with behavioral and learning problems.

- Molasses is a concentrated syrupy by-product of sugar cane or beet sugar refining. It is rich in nutrients such as B vitamins, vitamin E, iron, calcium, magnesium, potassium, chromium, manganese, and zinc. Molasses has a lower sucrose content than table sugar; the crude or blackstrap type is nutritionally preferable to sweeter varieties. Testimonials abound for the healing effects of molasses on disorders such as arthritis, anemia, ulcers, varicose veins, constipation, and low energy. Drawbacks to using molasses are similar to those associated with sucanat. Additionally, most brands are preserved with sulfur, high doses of which can be toxic. Tooth decay, hypo-glycemia, and diabetes can all be made worse by excessive use. Use unsulfured blackstrap molasses in moderation as you would sucanat.

- Sorghum molasses comes from a plant related to millet and looks like a dark syrup. It is rich in minerals such as potas-sium, iron, calcium, and the B vitamins. Its properties are sim-ilar to those of blackstrap molasses.

- Date sugar is more a food than a sweetener. It is made of ground-up dehydrated dates and is high in fiber and a long list of vitamins and minerals, including iron. Its use is limited by price and the fact that it does not dissolve when added to liquids. In small amounts, this is an acceptable substitute for sugar.

- Demerara sugar (raw sugar) is a granulated, dark brown sugar obtained from the evaporation of sugar cane juice. It retains some of the nutrients of raw cane sugar but is not as nutrient-rich as sucanat or molasses.

- Turbinado sugar is a further refinement of demerara sugar with fewer nutrients and more empty calories.

- Brown sugar is nothing more than ninety-one to ninety-six percent white sugar coated with molasses syrup and offers vir-tually no benefit beyond that of regular table sugar.

- Raw, unpasteurized honey is a good sugar alternative, but only because it is considerably sweeter and people tend to use less of it. Its composition is similar to that of table sugar, the major difference being a two-percent-higher amount of fructose than glucose (table sugar is fifty percent glucose and fifty per-cent fructose). Another advantage of honey over sugar is that it contains small amounts of vitamins and trace minerals, which vary from type to type. It is not, however, a good sugar substitute for either diabetics or hypoglycemics.

- Maple syrup is a naturally occurring sweetener which is, at the least, sixty-five percent sucrose. It is basically a sugar equivalent with a biochemical effect similar to that of raw, un-pasteurized honey. The greater expense of maple syrup is explained by the fact that it takes about forty gallons of sap from sugar maple trees to make one gallon of maple syrup.

• Barley malt is processed from cereal grains through enzymatic action and has the same total sugar content as maple syrup. Its properties are similar to those of brown rice syrup (see below), but the type of sugar is mainly maltose, which is less than half as sweet as sucrose. Since it is not as sweet as other sweeteners, there is a tendency to use more, which may be problematic in those with weight control or blood sugar problems. Barley malt is high in complex carbohydrates and enters the bloodstream slowly. It is less likely to upset blood sugar levels, but may still be problematic for diabetics and highly sensitive individuals. Barley malt contains some B vitamins and some trace minerals. Also, some individuals react negatively to it because MSG is often hidden in the malt.

• Fruit juice and rice syrup are commonly used as sweeteners in many health food store packaged cereals, cookies, and other products. Since both still contain sugar, albeit natural sugar containing some vitamins and minerals, they are still potentially a problem for diabetics and hypoglycemics. They are generally okay for healthy people provided that only small amounts are used (one to two servings daily of a cereal or box of cookies).

• Licorice root can be used as a natural sweetener in small amounts without serious adverse reactions. However, some extracts of licorice root, when used in large amounts or over the long term, can elevate blood pressure and cause water retention because they stimulate the adrenal gland. As a sweetener, licorice root is safe for diabetics or hypoglycemics, but *stevia* (see below) is preferred because it has no known side effects.

• Amazake is a natural disaccharide (double sugar) drink made from brown rice syrup. It can be consumed as a beverage or, in small amounts, used as a sweetener. Its characteristics are similar to those of honey or rice syrup, from which it is made. Brown rice syrup is a complex carbohydrate which enters the bloodstream more slowly than honey or maple syrup. Brown rice syrup contains some trace minerals and B vitamins, but at a lower level than barley malt syrup. It is less concentrated in flavor than other sweeteners.

• Fructooligosaccharides (FOSs) are sucrose molecules linked in sequence with fructose. They occur naturally in many vegetables, grains, and fruits. FOSs promote the growth of the beneficial gut bacteria (*lactobacillus acidophilus* and *bifidus*) and prevent fungal (candida) overgrowth. In Japan, FOS is used as a sweetener. Unfortunately, it is not broadly available in North America, and its use as a mainstream sweetener is inhibited by its current high price. Some health food stores sell FOS syrup for general sweetener purposes. A good natural source of FOS is Jerusalem artichoke flour. Other good sources include asparagus, onion, leek, garlic, dahlia inulin, chicory, and burdock. Burdock is part of the Essiac formula, which has been reported to have immune-boosting properties. The Essiac formula is made up of burdock, slippery elm, Turkish rhubarb, and sheep sorrel, four herbs with immune-boosting properties thought to be effective in cancer treatment.

Some of the other documented beneficial effects of FOS are a reduction of bowel toxins, the prevention of diarrhea and constipation, a reduction in serum cholesterol, the protection of liver function, and a lessening of chronic inflammatory bowel disease symptoms.

• *Stevia* is the name of a plant that has been used, in extract form, as a safe, natural sweetener by people in Paraguay and Brazil for hundreds of years. *Stevia* is two hundred to three hundred times sweeter than sugar. It has a slight licorice-like flavor that may take a little getting used to for some people. *Stevia* is virtually calorie-free, does not encourage cavities, and does not trigger a rise in blood sugar level. It does not nourish yeast, fungi, or other microorganisms in the gastrointestinal tract, but it increases energy level and improves digestion because of its ability to stimulate the pancreas.

Stevia is under attack by the U.S. Food and Drug Administration (FDA) and is being blocked from entering the country. However, domestically grown *stevia* is available in the United States. In 1991, the FDA banned the importation of *stevia* intended for use in foods. *Stevia* is many times cheaper than artificial sweeteners such as saccharine and aspartame. *Stevia* is also nonpatentable, another undesirable feature as far as the drug companies are concerned.

Artificial sweeteners are banned in Japan. Millions of Japanese consumers (more than forty percent of the sweetener market) have used *stevia*-sweetened products for the past two decades without any negative health effects. Dozens of well-designed studies of its safety, chemistry, and stability for use in food products have been published around the world. There has never been a report of an adverse reaction linked to the use of *stevia*.

Sugar alternatives: chemical sweeteners:

- Sucralose is an artificial sweetener with six hundred times the sweetening power of sugar. Not yet FDA-approved, it is legally in use in Canada and Australia under the brand name Splenda. There have so far been no reports of adverse effects, possibly because of its expense and limited use.

- Acesulfame-K (Ace-K) is a noncaloric synthetic sweetener composed of carbon, nitrogen, oxygen, hydrogen, sulfur, and potassium, approved in the United States in 1988 by the FDA. It is 200 times sweeter than sugar and more suitable than aspartame in cooking and baking because it retains its sweetness when heated. Ace-K is known for its bitter aftertaste, similar to that of saccharine. It is most often used in commercial products including baked goods, candies, and imitation dairy products.

- Cyclamates were banned in the United States by the FDA in 1970 because of their association with cancer. They have not, however, been banned in Canada, where, seemingly, people do not get cancer from them.

- Saccharine contains only $1/8$ calorie per teaspoon, is about three hundred times sweeter than sugar, and has a noticeably bitter aftertaste. Also associated with a cancer risk, in Canada it is only available from pharmacists. Saccharine is available in the United States pending further studies.

- Aspartame is still the king of the artificial sweeteners. It has a long history of controversy, with some authors and researchers calling it the most dangerous substance on the market.

  Aspartame causes over seventy-five percent of the adverse food-additive reactions reported to the FDA. Here are some of the ninety documented adverse effects of aspartame: headaches/migraines, dizziness, seizures, nausea, numbness, muscle spasms, weight gain, rashes, depression, fatigue, irritability, tachycardia, insomnia, vision problems, hearing loss, heart palpitations, breathing difficulties, asthma, anxiety attacks, slurred speech, loss of taste, tinnitus, vertigo, memory loss, and joint pain.

  Researchers and physicians report that many chronic illnesses can be triggered or worsened by aspartame. These include brain tumors, epilepsy, chronic fatigue syndrome, mental retardation, lymphoma, birth defects, fibromyalgia, and diabetes.

  According to research conducted by diabetologist Dr. H. J. Roberts, an authority on artificial sweeteners, aspartame can cause clinical diabetes, poorer diabetic control in diabetics on insulin or oral drugs, and aggravation of diabetic complications such as retinopathy, cataracts, neuropathy, and convulsions.

  According to Roberts:

  > Unfortunately, many patients in my practice, and others seen in consultation, developed serious metabolic, neurologic, and other complications that could be specifically attributed to using

aspartame products. This was evidenced by the loss of diabetic control, the intensification of hypoglycemia, the occurrence of presumed "insulin reactions" (including convulsions) that proved to be aspartame reactions, and the precipitation, aggravation, or simulation of diabetic complications (especially impaired vision and neuropathy) while using these products. Dramatic improvement of such conditions after avoiding aspartame, and the prompt predictable recurrence of these problems occurred when the patient resumed consuming aspartame products, knowingly or inadvertently.

Aspartame has been documented to cause low brain serotonin levels, depression, and other emotional disorders that are often reversed by stopping the use of aspartame. These results have been reported in people consuming as little as four sixteen-ounce bottles of diet soda per day.

Sweetener recommendations: Based on the available information from unbiased sources, it is clear that the healthy choice to make when it comes to sweeteners is to use only those from the natural category. Diabetics, hypoglycemics, and children suffering from candidiasis are best off using *stevia* or FOS as their mainstays and licorice root in moderation for healthy sweetening.

There is insufficient evidence of safety at the present time for any of the artificial sweeteners, especially aspartame. Until the FDA and HPB can adequately respond to the research done by Roberts and others, my advice can only be that aspartame and other chemical sweeteners should be avoided. For more action in this area, contact *Free World News,* My Health, My Rights, or the Alternative Therapies Health Association (ATHA).

Conclusion

In expanding the traditional view of childhood allergies, the door opens to new opportunities for parents and their children to both reverse and prevent chronic childhood illnesses. Food and chemical allergies include both immediate and delayed reactions, while chemicals that are responsible for a great deal of childhood illnesses go well beyond just drugs and MSG (monosodium glutamate). Chemicals such as chlorine and pathogenic organisms like *cryptosporidium* in tap water, as well as the thousands of unnatural additives contained in a child's food intake, can all have a direct impact on his or her health. Identifying and eliminating the majority of known allergens, be they the most commonly eaten foods or chemicals, can sometimes make all the difference in the world with respect to the incidence of many chronic or recurrent childhood illnesses.

As you will read in later chapters, children do not have to live with the daily need to take drugs for asthma, hyperactivity, recurrent ear infections, and other diseases. For many children, there are better, more natural alternatives. For other, more severe cases, the use of drugs can be reduced. In all cases, the information contained in this chapter provides both parents and doctors with the basic groundwork for a new and different approach to childhood illness. For example, knowing that relationships exist between commonly eaten foods, a high sugar intake, chlorine in the water supply, and eczema allows parents and their doctors to take more control over the triggers of recurrent health problems *like* eczema. The same can be said for a long list of child health issues to be discussed in the chapters which follow.

2 Testing for Allergies and Related Problems

Allergy Testing: Fact and Fiction

To understand which types of tests are valid and reliable in determining food and chemical allergies in children, it is important to realize that there are basically only two kinds of adverse reactions: delayed and immediate. Unfortunately, this concept is still not firmly grasped by the majority of the population, conventional allergists, and pediatricians.

The following is basic scientific information:

Immediate (type I) reactions:

- produce allergic symptoms (e.g., wheezing, swelling, choking, pain) that commonly occur two hours or less after consumption of the offending foods or chemicals; the food or chemical reaction is usually well known to the parent or child

- involve only one or two foods, for a given person, that cause allergic signs and symptoms (usually severe); these are the well-known, often life-threatening reactions to peanuts, shellfish, and strawberries

- are triggered by even trace amounts of allergenic foods or chemicals; it may take only the odor of cooked lobster to elicit intense allergic reactions (including anaphylaxis) in sensitive individuals

- are common in children and rare in adults

- are usually caused by a permanent or "fixed" allergy; these food reactions can be lessened by vitamin, mineral, and herb supplementation

- are associated with the IgE family of antibodies and can be verified by a skin test or a blood test called the IgE RAST (Radio-Allergo-Sorbent-Tests)

Delayed (type II, III, and IV) reactions:

- usually occur within twenty-four hours, and sometimes up to four days, after consumption of the offending foods or chemicals
- involve three to twenty foods that cause allergic signs and symptoms which are usually chronic (joint and muscle pain, fatigue, depression, psoriasis, etc.) and are hidden or unsuspected by the victim
- occur after larger amounts of foods are consumed (or chemicals inhaled), often in multiple feedings (or exposures); a single food or chemical challenge might not cause any allergic reactions
- are very common in children and adults; more than fifty medical conditions and two hundred symptoms are triggered, worsened, or caused by the allergic reactions
- are usually reversible within three to six months by a combination of food elimination and nutritional supplement therapy (antioxidants, enzymes, herbs, etc.)
- are not associated with the IgE family of antibodies but could be related to antibodies from immune complexes that involve antigen, antibody, and the inflammatory chemical called "complement" (type III reactions), or to cell-mediated immunity (type IV reactions); these types of reactions can be verified by blood tests

Most food-allergic people are unaware of their food allergies because, in a delayed reaction, the symptoms may occur many hours or days after ingestion. To further complicate things, if an allergenic food has not been eaten for several months and is accidentally ingested, a reaction may happen fairly quickly. For example, a child who is allergic to milk feels temporarily better each time he or she drinks milk. When the child stops drinking milk, he or she might initially feel worse for several days but, usually within seven to ten days, starts feeling better. After avoiding dairy products for six weeks, a large serving of milk may cause symptoms to be dramatically reproduced (wheezing, coughing, runny nose, irritability, etc.).

Delayed food allergies often create a complex blend of symptom-masking effects, withdrawal reactions, and symptom reproduction upon food reintroduction. Children with food allergies can behave as if they were addicted to foods. For example, a reaction to being withdrawn from milk can be stopped or lessened by a second glass of milk. This is the same thing that happens to the alcoholic's unpleasant withdrawal symptoms when given another glass of whiskey. Children often crave the foods that cause their symptoms; this is one fairly reliable way of knowing what should be taken out of their diets to improve their immune status.

Sorting Out the Confusion

Since over ninety percent of all food allergies are of the delayed-onset type, skin tests and the IgE RAST will not detect the vast majority of food allergies. Nevertheless, conventional doctors continue to use them for that purpose and often conclude that the patient "does not have any food allergies," even though no tests were ever done for delayed-hypersensitivity food reactions. For this and other reasons, those suffering from asthma, chronic sinusitis, hay fever, recurrent respiratory tract infections, and other diseases are told that food allergies have nothing to do with their illness and that only a lifetime of steroid, antibiotic, and antihistamine drugs will help.

There are many reliable tests that help detect food and chemical reactions. Although considerable confusion exists about which is the best laboratory test, most agree with the accuracy and reliability of the elimination-provocation technique described by food allergy pioneers such as Drs. William Crook and

Doris Rapp. This technique involves eliminating whole classes of foods for several days, then adding them back and observing reactions.

Workable variations of this include the Coca Pulse Test, which does not require a practitioner. The Pulse Test, developed by Dr. Arthur F. Coca, works as follows: Check the person's pulse just before eating a "suspected" food. Have your child eat the food, and recheck the pulse every thirty minutes for one hour. If the pulse rate has increased by fifteen or more beats within the next hour, and the increase can't be traced to exertion or an emotional change, a food allergy is indicated.

Another method of testing for food or chemical allergies is sublingual food challenges, which are usually administered by practitioners of environmental medicine. Some of these procedures would not be appropriate for children suffering from severe pain syndromes or for those who do not have the time or stamina to experiment with their diets. On the other hand, the elimination-provocation technique ultimately empowers sufferers to control symptoms with simple diet changes.

The Elimination-Provocation Test

The basic procedure in this food allergy test is to follow a hypoallergenic diet for three weeks, eliminating the most common food allergens, and thereafter challenge the body with the eliminated foods one by one and note the reactions. During the three-week elimination-diet period, symptoms (wheezing, runny nose, etc.) lessen in the majority of children who suffer from food allergies. If the reintroduction of certain foods causes a reproduction of the symptoms, the child is probably allergic to those foods. This diet works only if all the foods to be discontinued are eliminated abruptly, or "cold turkey." Easing into this diet slowly, or attempting some other compromise, does not work nearly as well because even minute amounts of an allergen stimulate the immune system to initiate reactions that lead to chronic symptoms.

In severely ill children (children with cancer, heart disease, brittle juvenile diabetes, cortisone-dependent asthma, or other life-threatening problems), it is not recommended that this approach be tried without close supervision by a medical doctor. Use common sense and the advice of your naturopath or doctor before attempting this on your own with your child. A sample elimination diet showing foods that a child can eat daily is found in Appendix II.

Foods to eliminate: Some foods and beverages should be eliminated regardless of suspected allergies because of their harmful effects on health in general. These are: all foods containing sugar, white flour, caffeine, chocolate, alcohol, hydrogenated fats (margarine, fried foods), and food additives of many kinds.

• Alcohol: found commonly in herbal and homeopathic tinctures and some prescription liquids (replace with non-alcoholic equivalents)

• Beef and pork: burgers, steaks, hot dogs, and cold cuts contain chemicals, additives, drugs, hormones, and carcinogens too numerous to list

• Caffeine: colas, soft drinks, chocolates, coffee, tea

• Citrus: oranges, lemons, limes, grapefruits, tangerines, mandarin oranges

• Corn: anything with corn oil, vegetable oil, margarine, corn syrup, corn sweeteners, dextrose, glucose, popcorn, tortillas, corn chips (read labels; "vegetable oil" usually refers to corn oil)

• Dairy products: milk, cheese, butter, yogurt, ice cream, sour cream, cottage cheese; read labels carefully because casein (milk protein), whey, caseinate, or anything containing these are dairy products and are even found in some soy-based products sold commercially; most margarines contain both corn and casein

• Eggs: both whites and yolks and anything made with eggs, such as quiche, French bread, pancakes, waffles, and egg substitutes

• Food additives: processed, packaged, and canned foods containing artificial colors, flavorings, preservatives, texturing agents, artificial sweeteners, or sulfites

• Known allergens: any foods known to produce symptoms (e.g., peanuts causing respiratory distress); do not eat any known reaction-producing food just because it does not appear on this list

• Seeds and nuts: most have high mold content, peroxidized fats, and other associated allergy problems; raw almonds, walnuts, sesame, and their nut butters are exceptions, but only for those children known to have had no reactions to them

• Sugar in any form: table sugar, candies, candy bars, cookies, pies, cakes, biscuits, sucrose, glucose, dextrose, corn syrup, fructose, maltose, levulose; pure, unprocessed honey, maple syrup, or barley malt in small amounts (one to three teaspoons) daily is allowed in some children at the discretion of the family doctor or pediatrician; avoid dried fruit because of mold and other additive content which could evoke allergic reactions

• Tap water: contains many chemicals, including chlorine, fluoride, and toxic heavy metals, and sometimes parasites; use distilled or mineral water sold in glass, not plastic, bottles; water treated by reverse-osmosis home filtration equipment is acceptable

• Vitamin and mineral supplements: only those without wheat, corn, yeast, and other additives are permitted

• Wheat: most pastas, breads, baked goods, cereals, semolina, durum, gravies, spelt, pizza (read labels; "flour" usually means wheat)

Foods permitted: Vary the diet as much as possible because one can become allergic to foods eaten too often, especially those eaten on a daily basis.

- Beans (legumes): kidney beans, lima beans, black beans, soybeans, tofu, lentils, chickpeas, green peas, string beans; soak all dried beans overnight, pour off the water, and rinse the beans before cooking; read labels for additives or prohibited foods if using canned beans

- Cereals: oatmeal, oat bran, puffed rice, millet; use soy milk, almond milk, or rice milk that has no corn oil or casein added; these types of products are found in many health food stores or grocery stores; diluted apple juice also works

- Fish, poultry, and fowl: trout, salmon, halibut, cod, shark, swordfish, mackerel, herring, tuna, sole, turkey, and chicken are good protein sources if they are from an organic "free range" source and packed in spring water if canned; canned shellfish (lobster, crab, shrimp) contain sulfites and other additives unless noted otherwise on the label

- Fruit: all except citrus and dried fruits, ideally from an organic source

- Grains: rice cakes, rye crackers (read labels because many rye products contain wheat), buckwheat Soba noodles, amaranth, quinoa; flours made from rice, potato, buckwheat, or beans; avoid spelt due to its similarity to wheat

- Lamb: hypoallergenic for most children

- Spices, condiments, miscellaneous: sea salt and pepper in moderation are acceptable; sugar-free ketchup, garlic, onions, kelp powder, wheat-free tamari sauce, cayenne, curry, and any other pure herbs in powder form known not to produce allergic reactions

- Vegetables: all are permitted except corn; ideal vegetables are from an organic source

Controlling elimination-diet problems: While following this diet, a small amount of weight loss may occur in the first week, as the fluid retained by the body in reaction to the allergenic foods leaves the system. The lost weight is temporary and not a problem, provided calories are also not restricted. If not enough of the permitted food is eaten, low blood sugar symptoms can develop. These include irritability, headaches, behavior problems, fatigue, and lightheadedness.

Withdrawal reactions occur in about twenty-five percent of people within a few days of starting the elimination diet. Some common withdrawal reaction symptoms are: flu-like illness, fatigue, headaches, a ravenous appetite, temper tantrums, and other behavior abnormalities. In most cases, these symptoms disappear within five days. If withdrawal symptoms are too severe to tolerate, antidotes one can use instead of giving in to the cravings are buffered vitamin C powder and bicarbonate powder (ideally one containing a mixture of potassium, sodium, calcium, and magnesium bicarbonate). Watch for diarrhea. If it occurs, reduce the dose until the antidotes can be tolerated. It's always best to discuss specific doses for your child with a natural health care practitioner.

How to test individual foods: Three weeks after continuing to follow the elimination diet, testing of individual foods can be attempted, provided that symptoms have either improved substantially or disappeared. If this did not happen, it is possible that the diet was incorrectly followed or that some allergic food or foods not on the list were eaten. In such cases, if food allergies are still suspected, alternative testing is more appropriate.

Only pure food from organic sources should be tested. For example, do not use a chocolate bar to test for chocolate, since chocolate bars are composites of dairy, wheat, corn, and dozens of other foods and chemicals. Only one food per day should be tested in relatively large amounts. If the reintroduction of foods reproduces the symptoms, the child is probably allergic to those foods. If headaches, fatigue, nasal congestion, upset stomach, joint pains, or other symptoms are caused by the food in question, it should be eliminated from the diet for at least six months.

In cases of autoimmune diseases such as juvenile rheumatoid arthritis, it is better to test foods every forty-eight hours because of the delayed reaction to foods so often seen in these disorders. In testing, if one is not sure whether there was a positive reaction to a specific food, keep it out of the diet and retest it in about a week. Testing foods the child never eats is unnecessary, as is testing for known food allergies.

Recommendations: Once you and your health care practitioner have established the most likely food allergens, these and anything containing them are eliminated while everything else eaten is put in a four-day rotation. A four-day rotation diet is one in which no food is eaten more than once every four days.

Foods that one is not allergic to can develop into allergens if they are eaten daily. For example, dairy-allergic children who go off milk, cheese, and other dairy products, then substitute soy milk and other soy products and consume them on a daily basis, eventually become allergic to soy products. A four-day rotation diet prevents this phenomenon.

After six to twelve months, the allergenic foods can be retested. If no reactions are noted, these foods can be eaten once every four days along with the other permitted foods. If there is still an allergic reaction, the food is kept out of the diet for another six months.

There are many variations of four-day rotation diets; one example is provided in Appendix II of this book.

Other Allergy Tests

There are no conclusive studies comparing the accuracy and reliability of different types of food allergy/sensitivity tests. Muscle testing and electro-acupuncture tests such as VEGA and Interro, combined with the subject's personal experience with different foods and professional counseling, have been documented to improve the lives of thousands. A VEGA test is one in which the subject's acupuncture points (which are part of his or her bodily electromagnetic acupuncture system) are tested for electronic disturbance patterns while the patient is holding various foods. A disturbance pattern on the VEGA machine indicates a physical reaction to the food in question. The Interro test is similar to the VEGA test, but it uses a computer programmed with the food to detect allergenic foods. Acupuncture and homeopathic diagnoses work for a great majority of people, but there are those who do not benefit from any aspect of these methods. The same can be said for various in vitro tests such as the Cytotoxic test and the RAST, FICA, and ELISA blood tests. However, the standard skin-scratch tests fail to detect the correct food sensitivities— scratch tests fail to detect fifty percent of food allergies and can also incorrectly identify a substance as an allergen.

The elimination-provocation test, when appropriate, combined with the ELISA/Act test developed by Dr. Russell Jaffe, is currently state-of-the-art in detecting hidden food allergies. The ELISA/Act test is a blood test which measures the presence of antibodies and white blood cell reactions to foods. If levels of antibodies are high or white blood cells react abnormally, the food tested is considered to be an allergen for that person.

The advantage of the ELISA/Act test is that it is capable of detecting delayed food allergies belonging to all of the delayed-reaction subgroups (type II, III, and IV reactions). It also measures any abnormal white blood cell reactions to specific foods. The ELISA/Act test can determine hidden or unsuspected allergies to as many as three hundred foods, chemicals, candida, mercury, and other toxic heavy metals. (For more information on the ELISA/Act test and doctors in your area who can order it, see Appendix IV.) RAST and FICA tests, offered by a large number of laboratories in the United States, rarely identify more than one hundred allergens and do not detect food allergies belonging to all of the delayed-reaction subgroups.

Much of the appeal of the blood tests for food allergies is the convenience of obtaining test results without going through the rigors of an elimination diet. The disadvantage of the blood tests is the cost (from $100 to $1,200, depending on the number of foods tested and the lab and physician fees). While more and more health insurance companies are providing coverage for the blood tests, many doctors still have concerns about the reliability of this form of testing for hidden food allergies. Although blood testing for food allergies has improved considerably over the years, different types of blood testing (IgE RAST vs. FICA, etc.) done on the same patient still yield different results in an unacceptable number of cases. Blood tests also cannot predict whether a specific food will produce the symptoms if consumed by the child.

In the future, with more research, time, and practitioner experience, the issues surrounding test validity and reliability will become clearer. In the meantime, children who eliminate offending foods from their diets reduce the allergic load on their immune system. This gives the body the opportunity to repair damaged tissues such as the joints, muscles, or lining of the respiratory tract. Those who are allergic to dust, ragweed, pollens, and other inhalant allergies can then be more tolerant to environmental allergens and less likely to suffer from severe allergic reactions that previously needed strong drugs for control.

Diagnosing Low Stomach Acidity

A mineral analysis of a child's (or adult's) hair can be used to determine excesses of toxic minerals or deficiencies of nutritional minerals. Natural health care practitioners are the best sources of testing. If hair analysis indicates an overall pattern of multiple low minerals, one might be in need of more acid to enhance the digestion and absorption of nutrients. It is rare for copper, zinc, and manganese levels to be low in an individual who takes appropriate nutritional supplements unless stomach acidity is low.

A high percentage of asthmatic and chronically ill children have low levels of stomach acidity. Low stomach acidity causes malabsorption of vitamin B-12 and a long list of minerals and amino acids. Low or absent hydrochloric acid levels can be confirmed by a CDSA (comprehensive digestive and stool analysis) test, performed by a naturopath or a medical doctor. (For more information on the CDSA, ask your practitioner to contact Great

Smokies Diagnostic Laboratory. There is also a lot of information on this type of test in both of my books, *The Joy of Health* and *Return to the Joy of Health.*) Low hydrochloric acid or digestive enzyme deficiencies can also be confirmed by a live-cell blood analysis. This is a special test done by high-magnification microscopy. Some naturopaths and doctors perform this test in their offices.

A lack (achlorhydria) or insufficiency (hypochlorhydria) of hydrochloric acid production by the stomach predisposes an individual to candida, fungal, parasite, or bacterial overgrowth. In normal, healthy individuals, the high acid content of the gastric juices will help kill off most fungi and other potentially harmful microorganisms found in food. Some of the major inhibitors of hydrochloric acid production are food allergies, especially to wheat, milk, and other dairy products. The problem can be reversed by eliminating the offending allergic foods and by supplementing the diet with acidifying nutritional supplements. Betaine and pepsin hydrochloride, as well as other stomach acidifiers such as glutamic acid and stomach bitters, dissolve candida and other microbes in the stomach. Excess acid, however, can cause severe heartburn and possibly lead to either gastritis or peptic ulcer disease. The need for acid supplementation should be determined by tests ordered by a natural health care practitioner.

Additional Tests to Determine Allergy-Related Conditions

Comprehensive Digestive Stool Analysis (CDSA)

The CDSA is done by collecting one or more stool samples, which are analyzed to indicate the body's ability to process food. The test checks for digestion and nutrient absorption problems, as well as bacteria, yeast, and fungi. It is especially recommended for children with chronic illnesses and those with a family history of cancer, inflammatory bowel disease, and autoimmune diseases.

The CDSA can help identify factors that contribute to leaky gut syndrome, such as enzyme and hydrochloric acid deficiencies and imbalances in the intestinal microflora. It can help direct natural health care practitioners to optimal nutritional intervention and supplementation.

Comprehensive Parasitology (CP) Test

Parasite infections can damage the bowel wall and deplete secretory IgA—the gut's immune system. The CP is another stool test usually ordered if one suspects the existence of parasites and their effects on the immune system via food allergies and the leaky gut syndrome.

Live-Cell Microscopy (LM)

Live-cell microscopy, also known as live blood analysis, or dark-field microscopy, is not a diagnostic procedure for any specific disease. It is best used as a screening test to help determine the optimal diet and natural therapies (enzymes, herbs, antioxidants, etc.) for a child with a chronic illness, especially a disease of the immune system.

Live-cell microscopy can show:

- abnormalities associated with hormonal imbalances
- abnormal blood clotting
- atherosclerotic plaque
- bacteria
- candida, yeast, fungi
- cell size and shape abnormalities associated with immune disorders
- digestive enzyme and hydrochloric acid deficiencies

- folic acid and vitamin B-12 deficiencies
- free radical damage
- iron deficiency
- parasites
- poor circulation and oxygenation levels
- undigested protein and fat
- uric acid crystals

Live-cell blood analysis differs from regular blood analysis in that it uses whole, live blood (as opposed to parts of the blood), is unstained, and uses higher magnification. The phase-contrast (dark-field) technique allows the technician to see more than can be seen using a conventional microscope.

The main advantage of blood microscopy is that many nutritional imbalances can be detected before standard chemical blood tests show any abnormalities. Health problems can then be prevented by early nutritional intervention.

Live-cell analysis involves the use of a microscope attached to a high-quality color video camera which is connected to a color monitor and a video recorder. One drop of blood from a fingertip puncture can provide valuable information concerning the presence of parasites, candida, fungi, and bacteria. The results of LM testing are then correlated with other physical and biochemical tests.

The presence of bacteria, fungi, or parasites revealed by LM should be used as a signal to take action by using natural antimicrobial therapies such as plant enzymes, echinacea, acidophilus, aloe vera juice, and green superfoods (spirulina and other natural immune system enhancers). Such steps can decrease the likelihood of infections and chronic illnesses developing.

3 Childhood Allergies and Nutrition

Food Families and Cross-Reactions

If one is allergic to a given food, one must avoid all foods within the same family in order to prevent adverse food reactions. Knowledge of food families is important for anyone who has food allergies. A person may be allergic to peanuts but tolerate almonds well. The opposite may also be true. The peanut is not a true nut but a legume in the same family of foods as lentils, lima beans, soybeans, and peas. A person with an allergy to peanuts may react adversely to lima beans or other members of this food family because they are related chemically.

Food Families

Apple: apple, pear, quince

Aster: lettuce, chicory, endive, escarole, dandelion, sunflower, tarragon

Banana: banana, plantain, arrowroot

Beech: chestnut

Beet: beet, spinach, chard

Bird: chicken, turkey, duck, goose, guinea, pigeon, quail, pheasant, other fowl, game birds, and their eggs

Blueberry: blueberry, huckleberry, cranberry, wintergreen

Borage: comfrey, fennel, borage oil

Bovid: milk, butter, cheese, yogurt, margarine, beef, lamb

Buckwheat: buckwheat, rhubarb

Cashew: cashew, pistachio, mango

Citrus: lemon, orange, grapefruit, lime, tangerine, kumquat, citron

Conifer: pine nut

Crustacean: crab, crayfish, lobster, prawn, shrimp

Flax, flaxseed, and flaxseed oil

Freshwater fish: sturgeon, salmon, bass, perch

Fungus: mushrooms and all yeasts, including brewer's yeast

Gooseberry: currant, gooseberry

Grape: grapes, raisins

Grass (grains): wheat, corn, rice, oats, barley, rye, wild rice, cane, millet, sorghum, bamboo sprouts

Honeysuckle: elderberry

Laurel: avocado, cinnamon, bay leaf, sassafras, cassia buds or bark

Legume: peanuts, peas, black-eyed peas, green beans, kidney beans, pinto beans, string beans, mung beans, navy beans, chickpeas, carob, soybeans, lentils, licorice, alfalfa

Lily: onion, garlic, asparagus, chives, leeks

Mallow: okra, cottonseed

Melon: watermelon, cucumber, cantaloupe, squash, zucchini, pumpkin, other melons

Mollusks: abalone, snails, squid, clams, mussels, oysters, scallops

Mulberry: mulberry, figs

Mustard: mustard, turnip, radish, horseradish, watercress, cabbage, broccoli, cauliflower, brussels sprouts, kale, kohlrabi, rutabaga

Olive: black or green olives

Orchid: vanilla

Palm: coconut, dates, date sugar

Parsley: carrots, parsnips, celery, celery seed, celeriac, anise, dill, fennel, cumin, parsley, coriander, caraway

Pawpaws: pawpaw, papaya, papain

Pedalium: sesame

Pepper: black and white pepper, peppercorn

Plum: plums, cherries, peaches, apricots, nectarines, almonds, wild cherries

Potato (nightshades): potato, tomato, eggplant, red and green peppers, chili pepper, paprika, cayenne, tobacco

Protea: macadamia nut

Rose: strawberries, raspberries, blackberries, loganberries, rose hips

Saltwater fish: herring, anchovy, cod, sea bass, sea trout, mackerel, tuna, swordfish, flounder, sole

Spurge: tapioca

Subucaya: Brazil nut

Swine: pork chops, bacon, ham, most cold cuts, hot dogs, sausages

Walnut: English walnuts, black walnuts, pecans, hickory nuts, butternuts

Yam: sweet potato and yam

Other Food Relationships

To further complicate matters, many foods that don't belong to the same family may cause "cross-reactions" because they are related in other ways. One example is the foods containing natural salicylates. Regardless of food family, anyone allergic to aspirin (acetylsalicylic acid) may need to avoid salicylate-containing foods such as apricots, blackberries, currants, grapes, limes, nectarines, peaches, plums, prunes, raspberries, raisins, and strawberries.

Many processed foods and beverages have salicylates added; these products should also be eliminated by anyone with a salicylate allergy. Foods in this category are ice cream, cake, jellies, jams, candy, soft drinks, dessert mixes, chewing gums, mint or wintergreen mouthwashes, toothpaste, and lozenges.

A person with a sensitivity to aspirin can also experience cross-reactions to tartrazine (FD&C Yellow No. 5) and sodium benzoate, so these are best avoided in foods, drugs, and cosmetics by such a person.

Some children are sensitive to some, but not all, components of common food allergens. For example, persons with a soybean allergy may react badly to soybean sprouts, tempeh, tofu, miso, soy sauce (both mold- and acid-hydrolyzed types), and hydrolyzed vegetable protein (HVP), yet tolerate soybean oil if it is free of soy protein.

Cross-reactivity also occurs strongly among kiwi, sesame seed, poppy seed, hazelnut, and rye. Sometimes cross-reactions occur between foods and environmental inhalants. For example, children who react adversely to pollen from trees such as alder, hazel, and oak may also react to eating hazelnuts.

Latex products have been reported to cause cross-reactions with avocado, banana, celery, chestnut, fig, papaya, passion fruit, and peach.

Introducing Foods to Children

Food allergies can be minimized or prevented if solid foods and beverages are introduced to the breast-fed infant properly. Some children are born with allergies due to in utero exposure. Parents should avoid giving infants cow's milk, wheat, oranges, eggs, and chocolate during the first year of their lives. After a year, it is best to introduce one new food at a time. A new food can be introduced every four days, watching for reactions such as sneezing, runny nose, rash, irritability, diarrhea, or vomiting. If any of these reactions occur, avoid giving the child the allergenic food thereafter. Ideally, well-tolerated foods should be rotated on a four-day basis to minimize the sensitization that often occurs when foods are eaten repetitively.

When they reach six months of age, breast-fed infants can be introduced to hypoallergenic puréed or mashed foods such as carrots, squash, broccoli, yams, sweet potatoes, cauliflower, Jerusalem artichokes, sprouts blended with water, kiwis, apricots, pears, cherries, peaches, grapes, bananas, and applesauce.

At nine months, parents can introduce cabbage, oatmeal, papayas, lima beans, string beans, potatoes, blackstrap molasses, split pea soup, millet, peas, and basmati rice.

At twelve months, children could be introduced to barley, tofu, parsnips, chard, asparagus, avocado, brown rice, garlic, onions, spirulina, and honey.

At eighteen months, children could start eating sesame, tahini, rutabaga, beans, lamb, green leafy vegetables, buckwheat, fish, eggplant, rye, chicken, beets, and kelp.

High-protein and highly allergenic foods should be introduced last, ideally after twenty-one months of age. These include eggs, turkey, beef, milk, citrus, wheat, corn, peanuts, high-yeast-containing foods, shellfish, and nuts not already listed.

Healthful Alternatives

When parents are advised to avoid feeding their children sugar, white flour products, and all foods containing additives, preservatives, and hydrogenated fats, the question most often asked is "What can my child eat?" (See page 67 for simple and practical solutions.)

Microwave Cooking

There is more to heating with microwaves than we've been led to believe. Recent research shows that microwave-oven-cooked food suffers severe molecular damage. Microwave radiation creates new compounds (radiolytic compounds) that are unfamiliar to our systems. Microwave heating can cause slight changes in infant formulas with a loss of some vitamins. Expressed human breast milk that is warmed in a microwave oven loses lysozyme activity and antibodies and fosters the growth of more potentially pathogenic bacteria. Whenever possible, use other forms of cooking than a microwave oven.

Vitamin and Mineral Supplements

Conventional medical science asserts that children only need the nutrients obtained from their food to maintain health. Although this may have been true in the past, numerous factors are now forcing us to realize that food supplementation is necessary if children are to attain optimal health.

Some of the things that have convinced me and many other nutritional doctors to recommend food supplements for children are:

1. Poor diets: Numerous published studies conclude that the quality of commercially available foods has declined greatly in

Replacing Harmful Foods with Healthful Foods

ELIMINATE:	REPLACE WITH:
sugar	molasses, honey, barley malt, rice syrup
salt	kelp powder, sea salt
potato chips	sourdough pretzels, rice cakes
beef/pork/veal	fish, lamb, wild game, soy products
salted nuts	fresh, unroasted almonds or macadamia nuts
white bread, rolls, buns, bagels	whole wheat bread, rolls, buns, bagels
white flour ("enriched")	whole-grain flours, bean flours
cookies, pastries, cake	whole fruits
donuts	whole-grain, low-fat muffins
commercial cereals	sugar-free granola, muesli, cooked grains
pancakes and waffles	whole-wheat French toast
white-flour tortillas	whole-wheat or corn tortillas
white crackers	whole-grain crackers
white flour pasta	whole-grain pasta from wheat, rice, corn
white rice	brown rice, wild rice, barley, quinoa
cow's milk	rice milk, soy milk, nut milk, amazake
cheese	tofu cheese slices and spreads
ice cream	frozen fruit, rice milk, soybean ice cream
margarine	ghee
popcorn with butter	air-popped popcorn with tamari and spices
peanut butter	almond or macadamia nut butter
commercial corn chips	baked corn tortillas
fried foods	broiled, poached, steamed, stewed, or baked foods
luncheon meat, canned meat	soy deli slices; bean, nut, or tofu spreads
hamburgers	soy/vegetable burgers, tempeh, falafel
ketchup	tomato sauce, sugar-free ketchup
vinegar	apple cider vinegar, lemon/lime juice

the past forty-five years. Studies on hospital patients and institutionalized children show that as many as eighty percent have one or more vitamin and mineral deficiencies. Studies indicate that the average North American is often deficient in vitamins A, B-2, and B-6, as well as the minerals calcium, magnesium, and iron. The situation may be even worse, since no studies have reported on nutritional analyses involving less well-known nutrients such as boron, silicon, inositol, biotin, and the three dozen or more other nutrients vital to health.

Studies show that well over fifty percent of children do not get even recommended daily allowance (RDA) levels of many nutrients. It is highly unlikely that any child in North America gets all of the necessary nutrients from the SAD (standard American diet). The majority of people eat processed, refined foods that lack fiber, vitamins, and minerals, and they tend to eat the same few foods over and over. Even the more conscientious, whole-food consumers without access to organically grown foods will not get all the nutrients they need from their food because of many factors that rob foods of vital nutrients. These include:

- chemical fertilizers

- pesticides

- herbicides

- transportation

- storage

- processing

- contamination with fungi

- packaging

- additives

- preservatives

Chemicals in the food supply (fertilizers, pesticides, herbicides, fungal contamination, additives, and preservatives) can create free radical reactions in the body that rob the body of its stores of antioxidant vitamins.

2. Poor digestion and absorption: Even if one eats a wide variety of organic foods, malnutrition can result because of an inability to digest and absorb foods properly. Millions of children have problems digesting, absorbing, and utilizing nutrients found even in the so-called well-balanced diet.

3. Personal stress, drugs, and pollutants: These factors can increase the need for certain nutrients such as vitamins A, C, and E, the B vitamins, calcium, magnesium, potassium, zinc, and essential amino acids. Nutrient reserves are used up and malabsorption results from weakened digestive cellular function. Surgery, prescription drugs, environmental pollution, and illnesses such as cancer further deplete nutrient reserves, even in the face of a high-quality "balanced" diet.

Some of the more commonly used drugs deplete important antistress vitamins and minerals. For example, aspirin can interfere with folic acid utilization and cause loss of iron from the body if used for extended periods of time. Dilantin and other anticonvulsants can lower the levels of vitamin B-12, folic acid, and other B complex vitamins. Antibiotics can interfere with the synthesis of biotin, vitamin B-12, and vitamin K because they destroy the friendly bacteria in the bowel responsible for digestion and vitamin production. Chlorine in tap water can deactivate vitamin C and many antioxidant enzyme systems in the body. Fluoride in tap water can paralyze numerous enzyme systems, depleting virtually all antioxidants (vitamins C and E, selenium, and others).

4. Physical stressors: Depletion of the protective ozone layer, air pollution, fluorescent lighting, noise, pollen, dust, dust mites, molds, and radiation (background and medical) all can cause higher levels of free radicals in the body, requiring additional antioxidant vitamins and minerals which may not be provided in sufficient amounts in the diet. Free radical production is

now thought to be one of the most important mechanisms by which diseases are created, and only free radical scavengers known as antioxidants will inactivate them. Free radicals are highly reactive, unstable molecules that possess unpaired electrons capable of disrupting cellular processes, leading to such things as bleeding, slow wound healing, secondary infection, pain, organ dysfunction, and chronic degenerative diseases (cancer, heart disease, arthritis, etc.). They are inactivated by antioxidants (certain vitamins, minerals, and enzymes). Few scientists now believe that even the best of diets can offer anyone enough of these free radical scavengers to prevent diseases such as cancer, autoimmune disorders, and allergies.

5. High levels of physical activity: Highly active children who participate in competitive sports require extra nutritional support—trace minerals, amino acids, and antioxidants—beyond what a well-balanced diet can provide. Physical stressors seen in sports of almost any kind can lead to musculoskeletal injury, infection, or exhaustion if nutrient levels in the body are not optimal. Supplementation is usually necessary to avoid free radical damage to the heart, lungs, and musculoskeletal and immune systems. Supplementation is discussed in more detail in Chapter 6.

The Best Supplements

The supplementation of vitamins, minerals, herbs, and other nutrients should be individualized as much as possible. People all have unique biochemical needs. The best way to sort out any confusion about vitamin and mineral supplements is to get some testing done. For the healthier child, a combination of blood, urine, and hair-mineral tests would be adequate. If there are symptoms of concern, a comprehensive digestive and stool analysis (CDSA) or live-cell microscopy would help identify hidden problems with digestion, absorption, free radical damage, or other signs of a need for supplements. Naturopaths and doctors interested in nutrition can order these tests for you or your child.

Most supplements are best taken with meals since this is how one would acquire them naturally in foods and beverages. Some amino acid supplements such as L-tryptophan are best taken on an empty stomach to avoid the influence of competitive amino acids for absorption into the system.

Live, whole-food concentrates have the unique advantage of supplying the body with enzymes and cancer-preventing phytochemicals such as carotenoids, indoles, isothiocyanates, isoflavones, and phytosterols which do not exist in any vitamin or mineral supplement. Additionally, they provide the body with amino acids, polypeptide hormone precursors, and other nutrients that support the vital life force needed by all cells for optimal health.

Using a whole-food supplement with the widest possible range of nutrients is preferable to just taking vitamin and mineral tablets. Examples of whole-food supplements are:

aloe vera juice (whole-leaf)

bee pollen

blue-green algae

chlorella

cruciferous vegetables (broccoli, cauliflower, brussels sprouts, etc.) as whole-food concentrates

desiccated liver

flaxseed, milled

garlic

green drinks or green food concentrates made from one or more of the following: alfalfa, blue-green algae, chlorella, chlorophyll, barley grass powder, green kamut powder, Japanese green tea extract, Jerusalem artichoke powder, spirulina, wheat grass powder, wheat sprouts

herbs

kelp, dulse, and other seaweeds

lecithin granules and other soybean derivatives

nutritional yeast

tissue concentrates (e.g., pancreatin, raw adrenal glandu-
lar concentrate)

wheat germ

wild yam extract

A combination of three or more of these (e.g., whole-leaf
aloe vera juice plus bee pollen plus a green drink) will provide
healthy individuals with all the vitamins, minerals, and enzymes
they might need for optimal health. Most children over age four
can supplement daily with a teaspoon of any of these mixed with
water or juice. Health care practitioners may recommend
specific combinations or higher dosages tailored to individual
biochemical needs. Eating a highly varied diet with plenty of
green vegetables, soy products, and other legumes should help
supply other vital nutrients. Some companies combine a large
number of whole foods, herbs, and accessory food factors into
one supplement.

Vitamin C

Vitamin C is important for the following reasons:

- it aids in formation of collagen and the health of bones, teeth,
  gums, nails, muscles, ligaments, and all other connective
  tissue;
- it strengthens blood vessels and prevents bleeding and plaque
  formation in the arteries;
- it promotes healing of all body cells;
- it increases resistance to infection;
- it aids iron absorption and utilization;

- it is an antioxidant that helps prevent cancer and heart disease;
- it is a natural antihistamine in high doses.

Vitamin C is best obtained from natural sources. If a child does not tolerate citrus, try peppers, garlic, onions, cantaloupe, kale, parsley, turnip greens, broccoli, rose hips, black currants, strawberries, apples, persimmons, guavas, acerola cherries, potatoes, cabbage, and tomatoes. All fresh fruits and vegetables contain vitamin C and varying amounts of bioflavonoids.

Signs of vitamin C deficiency: Worsening hay fever and bleeding gums are signs of vitamin C deficiency. They are also a sign of a greater need for bioflavonoids. Good examples of bioflavonoids include pycnogenol, quercetin, hesperidin, catechin, and rutin. These can be taken in high doses without side effects.

Recurrent nosebleeds (or bleeding from gums and other tissues) for no obvious reason also indicate a need for vitamin C and bioflavonoids, which are important for capillary and blood vessel wall integrity. The most effective bioflavonoids for nosebleeds are the proanthocyanidins (pycnogenols), of which grape-seed extract is considered to be the best. The dose that would be effective for most children under twelve is 100 to 200 mg daily for about three weeks, tapered down to about 50 mg daily thereafter for prevention. As for vitamin C, those with bowel problems should use either the buffered form of vitamin C or ester C (1,000 to 3,000 mg daily). Both vitamin C and bioflavonoids are also effective treatments for food, chemical, and environmental allergies.

Dealing with adverse reactions to vitamin C: Some children have bad reactions to vitamin C supplements, including headaches, gas, nausea, and lightheadedness. Often these symptoms can be overcome by using buffered forms of vitamin C such as sodium ascorbate, calcium ascorbate, ester C, and others. Bioflavonoids might also help improve the tolerance of vitamin C supplements.

Vitamin C is a weak acid. Candida, bacteria, fungi, and parasites are often killed off by high doses of vitamin C, and this releases toxins into the system. Gas, headaches, nausea, and lightheadedness sometimes result, but these are just signs of a temporary cleansing or detoxification reaction.

Buffered forms of vitamin C are needed when there are symptoms such as burning or pain after taking the pure ascorbic acid form. Headaches, nausea, gas, and dizziness that do not disappear within a few days of use also mean that a buffered form should be tried. Detoxification or cleansing reactions should dissipate in three to four days. If they worsen, excess acidity from too much vitamin C is probably the reason. Switch to a buffered form.

The problem can be eliminated by doing a "vitamin C flush." This involves increasing the dose of vitamin C to the point of producing clear, watery diarrhea and usually results in a nice purge of the majority of these toxins. The vitamin C flush is best done with buffered vitamin C powder, taking a teaspoon in juice every half hour until watery diarrhea occurs. After this bowel tolerance level is reached, the dose can be adjusted to where the bowels feel comfortable. Gas and other detoxification reactions should disappear.

If you do not wish to give your child a vitamin C flush, consider adding sodium bicarbonate to an ester C, sodium ascorbate, or calcium ascorbate supplement. This is available in powdered form and can be taken immediately after taking the vitamin C. Start with low doses and increase gradually as tolerated. Additionally, use a good *lactobacillus acidophilus* and *bifidus* supplement to help control the bowel flora, reduce gastrointestinal toxins, and improve digestion.

If your child has trouble tolerating even the buffered forms of vitamin C, consider getting her or him tested for chronic gastrointestinal dysbiosis. It is possible that there is a bacterial flora imbalance, candida overgrowth, bacterial infection, or parasites. A natural health care practitioner can order a CDSA with a comprehensive parasitology evaluation to rule out this potential problem.

Iron-Deficiency Signs and Symptoms

Symptoms of iron deficiency include fatigue and a lack of stamina. This is the result of fewer and paler red blood cells and a reduced ability of these cells to hold and carry oxygen. Iron deficiency in children has been reported to produce anemia, psychological problems, learning disabilities, hyperactivity, decreased attention span, and a lowered IQ. Other common iron-deficiency symptoms are headaches, dizziness, decreased appetite, weight loss, constipation, and weakened immunity. Anemia manifests itself as pallor of the skin, cheeks, lips, and tongue. Canker sores in the mouth, hair loss, brittle nails, and itching are other common symptoms.

People who suffer from iron deficiency will sometimes have unusual food cravings which promptly disappear after iron supplementation is successful. In children, iron deficiency may cause a strange symptom called "pica," a term that refers to the eating or chewing of nutritionless objects such as toys, clay, or ice. Iron treatment ends this behavior. Iron deficiency can be confirmed by blood tests, the most sensitive of which is the serum ferritin level. It might surprise you to know that the best sources of iron are vegetarian.

High Iron-Content Foods

Foods high in iron include:

- kelp
- brewer's yeast
- blackstrap molasses
- wheat bran
- pumpkin seeds

- whole sesame seeds
- wheat germ
- beef liver
- sunflower seeds
- millet
- parsley
- clams
- almonds
- dried prunes
- cashews
- lean beef
- raisins
- Brazil nuts
- pork
- eggs
- lamb
- chicken
- salmon

Combining Vitamins and Minerals

There are many misconceptions about whether one should take certain vitamins and minerals together. For example, it is often said that zinc and calcium cannot be taken together. In truth, all vitamins and minerals in the body work in cooperation with each other to catalyze enzymes and promote the absorption and assimilation of other vitamins and minerals. In other words, they work synergistically.

It is not a good idea to take a single vitamin or mineral supplement on its own. Although the toxicity potential of single-nutrient therapy is very low, one can optimize the effectiveness of any vitamin or mineral by considering some basic guidelines.

If a person is deficient in one vitamin, it is crucial to take a completely balanced vitamin and mineral preparation in addition to replacing the vitamin found to be deficient. For example, if you are giving your child long-term high doses of vitamin A for acne or vitamin C for fatigue, also give her or him a broad-spectrum multivitamin and mineral supplement as well as a whole-food supplement (see previous list) to prevent relative deficiencies in other nutrients.

There is no evidence that zinc and calcium cannot be taken together unless the supplements in question contain synthetic fillers, binders, and other unnatural ingredients. Some pharmaceutical brands of trace mineral supplements contain dyes, lactose, yeast, gluten, and other fillers that might inhibit absorption in some sensitive individuals. Stay away from these and look for brands that list all the ingredients on the label.

It is also often said that high-dose vitamin E supplements can interfere with iron absorption or vice versa. For doses of naturally occurring iron (15 to 18 mg daily), this is not an issue. But synthetic prescription iron doses (300 mg or more daily) produce problems, not only with constipation, but with the deactivation of vitamin E and other antioxidants. To avoid this as much as possible, use iron supplements about twelve hours apart from vitamin E.

Iron absorption is enhanced by sufficient acid in the stomach. A supplement of vitamin C (500 to 1,000 mg) can increase iron absorption by up to thirty percent. Other good iron absorption aids include stomach bitters, betaine or glutamic acid hydrochloride, apple cider vinegar, and lemon juice.

Dairy Products: Challenging Sacred Cows

Cow's milk is closely associated with "the American way." Parents have been conditioned to believe that milk and dairy products are vitally important parts of their children's diet. The National

Dairy Council spends millions of dollars annually promoting its products. Tradition, emotional attachment, and the marketing and advertising hype, reinforced by well-meaning pediatricians and family doctors, can be very convincing.

But cow's milk was created and designed by nature for calves, not infants or children. Consider the following dairy product facts:

• Milk contains sixty percent saturated fat (arachidonic acid) and is a major contributor to the development of atherosclerosis in young children.

• Milk is one of the most common food allergens in the North American diet for both children and adults. It is a major contributing factor in middle-ear infections (otitis media), gastroenteritis, anemia, asthma, eczema, headaches, juvenile rheumatoid arthritis, juvenile diabetes, bed-wetting, fatigue, hyperactivity, epilepsy, and recurrent respiratory infections of all kinds.

• Milk sugar (lactose) is indigestible by most of the world's population. Gas, cramps, bloating, and diarrhea might all be signs of an allergy to milk protein, or they could indicate a deficiency or a lower-than-optimal level of the enzyme lactase, which breaks down milk sugar.

• Milk prevents iron absorption and enhances the absorption of lead, a highly toxic mineral.

Even when allergy testing reveals that a child with recurrent middle-ear infections suffers from a severe allergy to dairy products, panicky parents and relatives find it difficult to eliminate dairy products because of worries about calcium and protein deficiencies and the social consequences. There is also a fear of criticism from the family doctor.

The value of cow's milk as a calcium source has been grossly exaggerated, notably by those connected to the dairy industry. Cow's milk has a high calcium content, but many studies demonstrate that absorption of the calcium in cow's milk is inferior to that of calcium from plant sources. For example, one recent study revealed that absorption of calcium from kale was 40.9 percent, compared with 32.1 percent absorption of calcium from cow's milk.

Recommended Sources of Calcium

Dark green leafy vegetables, with the exception of spinach due to its high concentration of oxalate, have relatively high calcium concentrations. Kale and other members of the same food family, such as broccoli, turnip greens, collard greens, and mustard greens, are also excellent sources of magnesium, a trace mineral that is important for calcium utilization and which is found in only small amounts in cow's milk.

In the past few years, several excellent green-food supplements high in both calcium and magnesium have come out on the market. These include spirulina, chlorella, barley green, green kamut, blue-green algae, and several others. These all make ideal supplements for children because they are easy to mix with juices, are easily absorbed, and have a good balance of dozens of trace minerals, antioxidants, vitamins, amino acids, and essential fatty acids.

The recommended daily calcium intakes for children are

infants: 360–600 mg/day

children: 800–1,200 mg/day

teens: 1,200 mg/day

Calcium Contents of Foods

GREEN LEAFY VEGETABLES:

collard greens	360 mg/cup
bok choy	250 mg/cup
kale	210 mg/cup
parsley	200 mg/cup
mustard greens	180 mg/cup
broccoli	160 mg/cup

(continues)

dandelion greens	150 mg/cup
chard	125 mg/cup
spinach	50 mg/cup
leaf or romaine lettuce	40 mg/cup

SEAWEED:

hijiki	350 mg/25 g
wakame	325 mg/25 g
arame	290 mg/25 g
kombu	200 mg/25 g

DAIRY PRODUCTS:

evaporated milk	635 mg/cup
goat milk	315 mg/cup
skim milk	300 mg/cup
buttermilk	300 mg/cup
whole milk	290 mg/cup
lowfat yogurt	270 mg/cup
whole-milk yogurt	250 mg/cup
cottage cheese	230 mg/cup
breast milk	80 mg/cup

BEANS AND PEAS (COOKED):

tofu	300 mg/cup
navy beans	140 mg/cup
soybeans	130 mg/cup
pinto beans	100 mg/cup
chickpeas	95 mg/cup
lima beans	60 mg/cup
lentils, kidney beans	50 mg/cup
split peas	20 mg/cup

SPROUTS (RAW):

soy	50 mg/cup
mung bean	35 mg/cup
alfalfa	25 mg/cup

FISH:

sardines with bones	370 mg/3 oz
salmon with bones	170 mg/3 oz
oysters	90 mg/3 oz

NUTS AND SEEDS:

sesame seeds	70 mg/tbsp
hazelnuts	25 mg/tbsp
tahini	20 mg/tbsp
pumpkin seeds	20 mg/tbsp
sunflower seeds	10 mg/tbsp

GRAINS:

corn tortillas	120 mg/2
quinoa	80 mg/cup
whole wheat flour	50 mg/cup
oats	40 mg/cup
dark rye flour	40 mg/cup
cornmeal	24 mg/cup
brown rice	20 mg/cup

OTHER:

blackstrap molasses	140 mg/tbsp

Calcium supplements: For children who need to get extra calcium from supplements due to a variety of problems such as food allergies, diarrhea, food availability problems, or malabsorption, the following possibilities could be considered:

- Calcium carbonate: has the highest amount of calcium per pill but may cause intestinal gas and/or constipation in susceptible individuals. If taken with meals or an acidifying supplement such as betaine, citric acid, or glutamic acid, absorption is enhanced.

- Calcium citrate: has less calcium per pill but is better absorbed than calcium carbonate and has no known side effects. This is the form of calcium most often recommended by health care practitioners.

* Calcium phosphate: is not recommended because excess phosphorus prevents calcium utilization. This is the form most commonly found in bone meal and inferior calcium supplements.

* Calcium lactate: is a reasonable supplement but should be avoided if one has dairy intolerance.

* Calcium gluconate: is a poor supplement which yields little, if any, calcium.

* Dolomite and bone meal: are not recommended because of questionable calcium absorption as well as contamination with lead.

Optimal bone development: Bone is active, living tissue continuously forming and being broken down. It is not just an inanimate collection of calcium crystals. The typical Western diet—high in refined carbohydrates, animal protein and fat, and canned and processed foods—has been linked to bone loss simply because such a diet is inadequate in a large number of nutrients. It is also excessively high in phosphorus, a mineral that, in large amounts, antagonizes calcium in the body. Interestingly enough, the foods most often recommended for healthy bones—milk and dairy products—are excessively high in phosphorus and actually promote bone loss.

The protein matrix upon which calcium crystallizes is called osteocalcin. Studies show that vitamin K is required by the body to make osteocalcin. Several other vitamins and minerals are important for bone health. Vitamin D is required for absorption of calcium from the small intestine. Deficiency can come about when there is reduced exposure to sunlight, decreased dietary intake, or a malabsorption problem. Other necessary nutrients include vitamin A, folic acid, vitamin B-6, vitamin B-12, vitamin C, magnesium, manganese, boron, strontium, silicon, zinc, and copper. Whole-food natural supplements containing all these nutrients include bee pollen, yeast supplements (nutritional yeast, brewer's yeast), and green drinks such as spirulina, chlorella, blue-green algae, and barley green.

Popular children's vitamins often do not contain most of the nutrients found in these products. For most healthy children age four to twelve a good broad-spectrum multivitamin and mineral supplement found at a health food store may be enough. Look for brands containing most of the ingredients discussed above. For children with bone or teeth problems, add silica gel, a green drink, and bee pollen to optimize bone growth.

High-protein diets, as well as a high intake of milk and other dairy products, encourage high mineral losses in the urine and actually prevent optimal bone development. This goes against the traditional "wisdom" of the dairy industry but has been verified by a great deal of published research. For more information on the deleterious effects of animal products and dairy products on bone development and health, read *Diet for a New America* and *May All Be Fed*, both by John Robbins.

Avoidance of sugar, refined carbohydrates, and processed foods is also important. Optimally, the diet should be high in fresh fruits, vegetables, whole grains, legumes, seeds, and nuts, all of which are high in not only calcium but dozens of other trace minerals. Regular exercise is also very important to boost bone growth.

Apple Cider Vinegar

Authors such as D. C. Jarvis, M. Hanssen, and C. Scott have written a great deal about the therapeutic effects of ingesting apple cider vinegar. Apple cider vinegar is made by fermenting the juice of whole, fresh apples. It is high in calcium, potassium, sodium, phosphorus, and other trace minerals. It has an average acetic acid content of five percent, and has been used both as a food and as a medicine.

Published research indicates that apple cider vinegar inhibits diarrhea due to its astringent property, helps oxygenate the blood, increases the metabolic rate, improves digestion, fights tooth decay and intestinal parasites, and improves blood clotting ability. It seems to also alleviate bad breath. In children, the value of apple cider vinegar is primarily as an acidifier. Asthma, autoimmune diseases, allergies, constipation, indigestion, and infections in children can be helped by this supplement. It can be mixed with salads and vegetable juices.

A long list of conditions can be improved by apple cider vinegar supplementation including obesity, infections, allergies, arthritis, fatigue, circulatory disorders, and thinning hair. Apple cider vinegar can increase the body's acidity, which produces a beneficial effect in many individuals. In others, the excess acidity makes their symptoms worse. Some children are allergic to apple cider vinegar, and in some cases it has no effect whatsoever. It's all a matter of biochemical individuality. The low toxicity and potentially spectacular health effects of apple cider vinegar make it well worth trying for those suffering from a wide range of suboptimal health conditions.

Plant-Based Diets

The number of children who follow a vegan diet (a vegetarian diet that also eliminates dairy products and eggs) has been growing in the past decade. While many parents are concerned about restricting their children's diets, provided calories are adequate, most nutrient needs, including protein, calcium, iron, and vitamin B-12 can be met by an entirely plant-based diet. The average American child gets four or more times the recommended amounts of protein from foods like hamburgers, peanut butter, cheese, and milk.

There are some children who are at risk for not getting the needed amount of protein from a vegan diet. Studies of vegetarian children show mixed results. Many children get all the protein they need, while others do not. The determining factor appears to be caloric intake. As long as a vegan child is getting enough calories, the protein need takes care of itself. If a child consumes dairy products and eggs on a regular basis, protein deficiency is certainly not an issue.

Vegetarians can run into problems if they rely too heavily on dairy products and wheat and do not eat a large variety of vegetables, fruits, legumes, and whole grains.

It is not true that those with a compromised intestinal lining (from celiac disease, colitis, Crohn's disease, etc.) should eat meat; a plant-based diet that is free of gluten, lactose, and sugar can be used with great success in the majority of these cases. Only a little imagination and extra effort are required to put together such a diet.

It is an established biochemical fact that all disease exists in an acid medium. All animal products, refined foods, and most grains create an acid condition in the body. Plant-based diets create more of an alkaline body pH. The meat-based, low-carbohydrate, or "caveman" diet advocated by many candida treatment gurus often does more harm than good because it creates an acid body pH and often results in a diseased state termed "ketosis." It is therefore not uncommon to see patients with celiac disease, Crohn's disease, or candidiasis who have been on long-term meat-based diets suffering from the side effects of excess acid: greater fatigue, weight loss, and dehydration. Also, a common symptom of candidiasis is constipation, a nuisance worsened by meat consumption.

One of the standard but erroneous criticisms of plant-based diets is their purported lack of iron. The best sources of iron are actually vegetarian. Another mistaken belief is that vitamin B-12 is only available in animal foods. Recent studies have shown that some sea vegetables contain substantial amounts of vitamin B-12, much more than enough to meet the nutritional needs of anyone. The sea vegetables include *arame, wakame,* and *kombu.* Others include *hijiki, alaria,* and *nori.* Tempeh, sauerkraut, pickles, and tamari also contain significant amounts of

B-12, as does miso if it is unpasteurized and prepared with traditional miso cultures. Vitamin B-12 is manufactured by the body's friendly colonic bacteria. Deficiency is most often related to poor absorption and an abnormally altered gut flora rather than a vegetarian diet.

For those who find sea vegetables and cultured soy products unpalatable or unavailable, I suggest the following natural food supplements that are rich in vitamin B-12: blue-green algae, chlorella, barley green, and spirulina. Supplementing with *lactobacillus acidophilus* is yet another way of getting vitamin B-12 into the body. All of these supplements are widely available at most health food stores.

The recommended daily allowance of vitamin B-12 is 2 mcg for infants and 3 mcg for children. Check the labels to make sure that your children are getting at least these levels from any food supplements.

Other than from cold-water fish, the majority of which are contaminated with either mercury or polysyllabic carcinogens, omega-3 fatty acids are best derived from plant sources such as flaxseed oil, seeds, nuts, and legumes. Omega-3 fatty acids have been proven to be effective in the prevention and treatment of many allergy-connected illnesses including asthma, rhinitis, eczema, migraines, and juvenile rheumatoid arthritis.

4 Childhood Allergies and Infection

Two children may be exposed to the same germ. One gets sick; the other remains well. Antoine Bechamp, a renowned French scientist, theorized that this phenomenon is due to the person's internal degree of friendliness toward the hostile microbes. If the body's biochemistry and immunology are sufficiently hostile to resist colonization by these potentially dangerous organisms, infection will not occur.

Though zapping such unfriendly microbes with antibiotics seems logical, a growing number of scientists and clinicians believe that it is much more important to improve or rebalance the child's internal environment to promote stronger resistance to viruses, bacteria, fungi, and parasites.

One way in which the internal environment can grow to favor infections is through poor nutrition in the form of a high-sugar, highly refined diet. Bacteria, fungi, and parasites flourish in a sugary environment. Another way in which children make it easy for pathogenic microbes to produce infections is to consume foods that cause adverse reactions. The majority of food and chemical allergies occur on a delayed basis and are hidden or unknown to the child and parent.

A delayed food allergy is most often from a commonly eaten food such as milk, wheat, corn, egg, yeast, chocolate, citrus, or soy. The allergic child's white blood cells can identify any of these as an invader and react by producing antibodies to break down and neutralize the food. When this happens over and over, weakened cell repair ability and damage to the white blood cells and organs can result. In the long term, the immune system can become preoccupied with fighting the "enemy" foods and less able to defend against viruses, bacteria, fungi, and parasites.

The common medical approach to recurrent infections is prescription antibiotics. While this treatment is certainly valid for serious infections, repeated courses of antibiotics alter the child's bacterial flora in the intestinal tract, encouraging the growth of fungi and candida. These organisms can secrete toxins which further weaken the immune system and increase the occurrence of both immediate and delayed allergic reactions. More drugs in the form of antihistamines, decongestants, steroid inhalers, and other allergy-suppressing treatments are prescribed, the infection rate accelerates, and more antibiotics are required.

The way to stop this vicious circle is to clean up the child's diet by eliminating sugar and refined and low-nutrition foods and to identify and eliminate foods to which the child is allergic.

Rising Infection Rates

According to the World Health Organization, nine million children die each year from infectious diseases. In the past twenty years alone, thirty new infectious diseases have appeared. Tuberculosis (TB) is making a comeback in parts of North America and is still the deadliest disease, infecting about one-third of the world's population and killing three million people each year. Malaria, dengue fever, AIDS, and the Ebola virus are just a few of the many new infectious diseases making the news. Increased world travel, human contact with previously uninhabited areas, overcrowded cities, and the misuse of prescription antibiotics, steroids, and hormones are a few of the reasons for rising infection rates.

In North America, sanitation is considerably better than in parts of the world where the Ebola virus causes epidemics. The major factors causing higher infection rates in North American children are increasing levels of environmental pollution, diets too high in sugar and additives, and the overuse of prescription antibiotics and other drugs. Infections such as otitis media, chronic fatigue syndrome, and respiratory tract infections—especially asthmatic bronchitis—are on the rise among North American children.

Antibiotics do not discriminate; they kill off friendly bacteria as well as the pathogenic ones in the intestines. Friendly bacteria such as *lactobacillus acidophilus* exist in the intestines to manufacture vitamins and to aid the digestion. When they are eradicated by antibiotics, the bowel can become colonized with unfriendly bacteria and fungi such as *Candida albicans,* which are not ordinarily found in large amounts in the bowels of healthy children. This results in long-term problems such as vitamin deficiencies, maldigestion, abnormal food reactions, malabsorption, gas, malnutrition, and tumor formation.

Antibiotics also cause allergic reactions, with symptoms such as diarrhea, rash, upset stomach, and candida overgrowth conditions (thrush and gastrointestinal dysfunction). With repetitive antibiotic prescriptions, many strains of bacteria become resistant to nearly all antibiotics in common use. This is worsened by the antibiotic residues in beef, pork, poultry, and dairy products.

Parents can prevent this tragedy from occurring in their children by making changes in general lifestyle factors: cleanliness, adequate rest, a nutritious diet, attention to adequate daily waste elimination, the provision of a nontoxic environment, optimal vitamin and mineral supplementation, the proper treatment of food and chemical allergies, and other means of naturally boosting immunity and wellness.

The Cure for the Common Cold and Flu

The flu (influenza) occurs in epidemics during late fall and winter, while a cold occurs anytime. Cold symptoms include sore throat, runny nose, aching, fever, headaches, and upper respiratory congestion. Flus usually develop quickly, are more severe, and involve fever, aching muscles, and acute fatigue. Most conventional doctors believe that the common cold and the flu are caused by exposure and susceptibility to common viruses. The truth is that not everyone exposed to these viruses develops a flu or cold.

Most natural health care practitioners believe that a cold is a cleansing attempt by the body to rid itself of waste overload. A child's immune response can become overwhelmed by a build-up of toxins resulting from fermentation, putrefaction, and the waste products of bacteria, fungi, and parasites. The immune system attempts to drain the body of excess mucus and toxins through coughing, a runny nose, sneezing, and sweat from a fever. Suppressing these symptoms with antihistamines, decongestants, and cough suppressants prevents the body from eliminating all the toxins.

The best treatment for the common cold is prevention. This involves avoiding food and chemical allergens and boosting immunity naturally. Not only can food allergies aggravate the signs and symptoms of a cold, but they predispose a child to become repeatedly infected with every bug that comes around. If a child with a healthy, functioning immune system does come down with a cold or flu, it should not last more than two or three days.

Good nutrition is the major means of prevention. This means reducing intake of all foods that decrease the immune system's functioning, especially simple sugars and sugar substitutes (cane sugar, corn syrup, honey, concentrated fruit sugar, aspartame). Within half an hour after ingestion, sugar suppresses the ability of white blood cells to function optimally.

Eliminate all foods that are difficult to digest and that are known to harbor bacteria, parasites, hormones, pesticides, or antibiotics. These include "junk" foods, red meats, poultry, and other animal products. Synthetic food additives (colors, sweeteners, artificial flavorings, preservatives, and oils) also suppress the immune system. High-protein foods such as meats, milk, eggs, and nuts, eaten in combination with highly concentrated carbohydrates such as fruit and other sweet foods, cause fermentation in the gastrointestinal tract leading to the development of even more toxins. Recurrent respiratory tract infections have been linked to the frequent ingestion of dairy products, wheat, artificial additives, and chemicals such as MSG.

A variety of herbal remedies work quite well to cure a cold or flu. These are bayberry bark, rose hips (which are high in vitamin C), white pine bark, white willow bark, cloves, capsicum, echinacea, goldenseal, calendula, astragalus, osha, and boneset. Zinc gluconate lozenges have also been reported to speed recovery from a flu or cold by soothing sore throats and healing canker sores and other oral cavity irritations.

Mucus elimination can be enhanced by consuming a green drink such as spirulina, chlorella, or blue-green algae. Drinking lots of purified water, herbal tea, and highly diluted fruit juice is also beneficial for speeding up mucus and toxin elimination.

Natural Treatment of Chronic Coughs

Chronic coughs that do not seem to be related to any specific medical illness are often caused by nutritional deficiencies and hidden allergies to foods or chemicals. A child with a chronic cough should be properly tested by a natural health care practitioner.

Meanwhile, the following natural remedies are good at both soothing a chronic throat irritation, settling down coughing spells, and preventing allergies of almost any kind from causing severe reactions:

- Vitamin A for short periods of time (two to three weeks) can be very soothing to inflamed mucous membranes. Vitamin A is also able to stimulate interferon (a natural immune system booster manufactured in the body by the white blood cells) production.

- Vitamin C and bioflavonoids, especially proanthocyanidins (pycnogenols from grape-seed, pine bark, or bilberry), quercetin, hesperidin, catechin, and others, are strong antioxidants which can both protect and heal mucous membranes. In order to derive any benefit from vitamin C treatment, one must push dosages up to bowel tolerance, the dose at which loose bowel movements are seen. For most children, this would be above 3,000 mg daily. Start with 3,000 mg and give 1,000 mg every four hours until bowel movements are loose. If bowel movements are not loose after twenty-four hours, double the dosage over the next twenty-four hours until the bowels are loose. The only significant side effect of taking vitamin C is diarrhea. Dosages should be reduced if the side effects become too uncomfortable. Besides chronic coughs, almost all viral conditions respond well to bowel-tolerance doses of vitamin C.

- Zinc gluconate lozenges are very effective against a chronic cough. One recent study of adults showed that taking about ten zinc lozenges (containing 23 mg of zinc each) per day reduced the length of recovery from the common cold from an average of 10.8 days to 3.9 days. Children between the ages of four and twelve can take approximately one-half this dose. Children under four can take about one-quarter of this dose. One of the reasons for the effectiveness of zinc is that it is a cofactor for a number of enzymes involved in the immune response. Zinc deficiency is associated with a compromised immune response and is normalized by zinc replacement therapy.

- Echinacea can also be used to treat chronic coughs. It has a reputation as a blood purifier and has been found to have interferon-like properties, making it an excellent immunity enhancer. Most herbalists recommend that echinacea be used on an intermittent basis—three weeks on, two weeks off—because its immune-boosting effects fail to occur if it is used continuously. Echinacea is best consumed as a tea or in a tincture.

- Goldenseal can also help a chronic cough. It has immune system–stimulating properties and is a potent activator of macrophages, which are cells that help gobble up bacteria, viruses, fungi, or other invaders.

- Licorice root can also soothe a chronic cough. It has been used by many cultures worldwide as a tonic, an energy booster, and a natural anti-inflammatory, as well as a natural antiallergy remedy. It has also been used to treat respiratory tract infections, congestion, hepatitis, Addison's disease, adrenal insufficiency, and digestive problems including ulcers. The two primary components of licorice—glycyrrhizin and glycyrrhetinic acid—stimulate the production of interferon by the body. Licorice heals inflamed mucous membranes in the respiratory tract and can be taken as a tea, tincture, or capsule. In large doses, licorice can cause high blood pressure in some sensitive individuals. For this reason, long-term use of licorice should be supervised by a naturopath or holistic medical doctor. In children, though, blood pressure problems are extremely rare.

- Astragalus is a well-known Chinese herb that enhances the antibody reaction to antigens that occur in allergies, infection, and cancer. Coughs of any kind respond well to it.

- Boneset is an herb that was used successfully by Native Americans for the treatment of chronic coughs, colds and flus, fevers, indigestion, and pain. It has antiseptic properties, promotes sweating, is antiviral, and boosts the immune system by enhancing the body's own secretion of interferon.

Herpes

Herpes is an annoying and occasionally serious viral disease easily recognized by most as a cold sore (type I). It can also occur anywhere in the genital area, where the blisters can be extremely painful and stubborn to heal (type II). Both type I and type II infections appear as blisters. Herpes is spread orally, by skin-to-skin contact, or through sexual activity. Conventional medical treatment is with drugs such as acyclovir (ointment and/or tablets), which can reduce the severity of attacks. I do not recommend it except in very rare cases.

Ultraviolet light can stimulate the reactivation of the herpes simplex virus under the skin. Application of a PABA sunscreen before going outdoors will help prevent sunlight-induced lesions. Beta carotene supplementation (100,000 IU or more daily) can also help block free radical sun damage for those who wish to prevent herpes outbreaks after spending time in the sun.

The mineral lithium may be of help to those who cannot tolerate acyclovir or other often prescribed antiviral drugs. Lithium interferes with the replication of the virus without affecting the host cells. It can be used in a topical ointment (8 percent lithium succinate) or combined with zinc (zinc sulfate solution 0.025 percent). Another potent, natural antiviral agent is colloidal silver, which can be taken internally or used topically without significant side effects. It is available through naturopaths and at health food stores.

Preventing Skin Infections

The health of the skin, the body's largest organ, may be dependent on stress, emotional factors, heredity, proper nutrition, the immune system (e.g., food and chemical allergies), and the digestive system, especially with respect to assimilation of nutrients and elimination of waste materials. Like the kidneys and the bowels, the skin excretes toxins present in the body. Impetigo or acnelike rashes are usually an attempt by the body to eliminate toxins that are not properly eliminated by the bowel.

To optimize skin health, the diet should be as natural as possible. Your child's diet should avoid chemicals, processed foods, high-fat junk foods, caffeine, alcohol, and sugar in any form other than fresh fruit. Animal products, including all dairy products and eggs, contain fats that can aggravate skin problems. They may also be loaded with drugs such as antibiotics, steroid hormones, nitrates, nitrites, and other toxins. Organic fruits, vegetables, whole grains, seeds, nuts, and legumes are best, provided one knows there are no allergies to these.

Healthy skin requires adequate amounts of water as well as many vitamins, minerals, enzymes, and other food factors. One of the most important groups of food factors is the essential fatty acids found in seeds (sesame, pumpkin), nuts (pine, walnut), and oils (flax, canola, evening primrose, olive).

Vitamins A, C, and E, beta carotene, zinc, copper, selenium, silicon, proanthocyanidins (pycnogenols such as pine-bark extract and grape-seed extract), and other antioxidants can prevent skin damage of any kind. In particular, they provide a greater degree of protection from sunburns, infections, and skin cancer. Antioxidants are also important in the healing process of any skin disorder or trauma including eczema, cuts, and abrasions. The fat-soluble vitamin D is also of great importance for skin health (from cod or halibut liver oil).

The amino acids, the B complex vitamins (especially biotin), and many other trace minerals are also important for the health of the skin. Good sources of these include green superfoods such as spirulina, chlorella, wheat grass, and herbs such as goldenseal, echinacea, red clover, and yellow dock. Aloe vera juice, bee pollen, Kombucha tea, *lactobacillus acidophilus,* and bifidobacteria all help provide the majority of nutrients required for healthy skin.

Some children develop deficiencies in these and other nutrients because of a number of digestive problems. The most common of these are low stomach acid, low pancreatic and intestinal enzyme levels, parasites, candida overgrowth, and bacterial flora imbalance in the large bowel. Live-cell analysis by phase-contrast or dark-field microscopy, as well as a CDSA, can be useful assessment tools for the presence of any of these potential hazards to optimal skin health. In severe cases, a good bowel detoxification program will be necessary. If possible, see a natural health care practitioner for more thorough biochemical and nutritional testing and a personalized treatment program.

Recurrent Middle-Ear Infections

Middle-ear infection affects two-thirds of children in the United States by the age of two and is the most common cause of acquired hearing loss in children. Allergies to milk and other common foods and the frequent and indiscriminate use of prescription antibiotics are at the root of most infections in children, especially middle-ear infections.

Fungal infections are the usual side effect of the use of pro-phylactic antibiotics. Fungi, through the production of mycotox-ins, may act as immunosuppressants, especially with respect to cellular immunity (the impairment of white cell defense against bacteria, viruses, parasites, etc.). This then leads to more ear infections, more antibiotic prescriptions, and so on. Antibiotics wipe out the friendly microbial flora in the gut, allowing candida and other fungi to multiply and damage the lining of the gut, leading to leaky gut syndrome, which then allows the absorption of food allergens. Furthermore, infants and children who are frequently prescribed antibiotics for middle-ear infections have been noted to have a much higher incidence of both hyperactiv-ity and autism.

Many researchers and authors, especially Dr. William Crook, believe that the epidemic of middle-ear infections in North America is a direct result of antibiotic-caused fungal infec-tions in the gastrointestinal tract. Often, the only way to break the vicious cycle is to treat the fungus with either natural or pre-scription remedies, or both, and to revise the diet by eliminating sugar, refined carbohydrates, and food allergens.

Before you decide on surgery to implant ear tubes for your children, take a look at their nutritional habits. Recent research suggests that food allergies may play a big role in recurrent otitis media, a condition that can sometimes lead to hearing loss. The top food allergens identified by researchers are cow's milk, wheat, egg whites, peanut products, soy, corn, and oranges. When children avoid those foods for four months, there is an eighty-six-percent improvement in the ears and hearing of children who had been advised to have ear tubes implanted. Both the frequency of the infections and the amount of fluid in the ears decrease significantly. When children add back the offending foods, ear infections return.

Food allergies are thought to increase fluid in the ear by creating nasal congestion; the fluid from the back of the nasal passages moves easily to the ear through the Eustachian tube, the passageway that connects the middle ear with the nose. When there is enough congestion in the Eustachian tube, it gets blocked and the fluid sits in the ear. Bacteria then start to multiply, and ear pain with fever eventually occurs.

Serous Otitis Media

Serous otitis media is the name given to a chronic, noninfectious inflammatory disease of the lining of the Eustachian tube, middle ear, and mastoid air cells. It can cause hearing impairment due to the recurrent accumulation of fluid behind the eardrum.

Serous otitis media is now estimated to affect ten million children in the United States and cost over two billion dollars each year. It is the most common reason for office visits to pediatricians and the most common disease seen by otolaryngologists (ear, nose, and throat specialists). Serous otitis media is the most common reason for pediatric surgery in the United States and England.

Conventional medical thought suggests that the serous accumulation of fluid could be the result of an unresolved or an inadequately treated acute otitis media. A second possible cause is an allergic predisposition to the condition. These mechanisms are not mutually exclusive, and both could contribute to or be caused by viral or bacterial infections. Testing for allergies, nutritional deficiencies, and other biochemical imbalances is certainly a good idea before resorting to surgical implantation of ear tubes.

5 | Additional Causes of the Childhood Illness– Allergy Connection

No one seems certain why the incidence of childhood allergies and the diseases arising from them are on the increase. Some say the overuse of antibiotics has a lot to do with it, while others point to the damage caused by vaccines, parasites, environmental pollution, prescription drugs, aspirin, and stress. This chapter examines some of these other childhood allergy associations.

Often, natural therapies will appear difficult and demanding to those used to conventional therapies. Explaining all possible causes with an open mind, however, may provide surprising—and welcome—results.

The Effects of Cigarette Smoke

Childhood illnesses and allergies are made worse by exposure to tobacco smoke. The evidence pointing to the hazards of secondhand cigarette smoke is overwhelming. Sidestream smoke contains far more carcinogenic tars and harmful particles than inhaled smoke which has passed through a cigarette filter.

A highly allergic child or one with lung disease suffers more seriously from cigarette smoke exposure than does an elite athlete, but both are likely to be adversely affected. The degree of danger also has to do with biochemical individuality. For example, some smokers and children who live with smokers live to a ripe old age, while others develop lung cancer at the age of thirty-five. It is to everyone's advantage to avoid secondhand smoke, but individual health circumstances will dictate how crucial it is to avoid it at all cost.

Exposure to secondhand smoke can produce a long list of acute symptoms including shortness of breath, asthma, pneumonia, bronchitis, headaches, fatigue, and irritation of the eyes, nose, throat, and lungs. Long-term exposure could lead to recurrent infections and chronic immune system problems such as allergies and autoimmune diseases.

Since tobacco smoke contains numerous carcinogens, exposure increases the risk of cancer. According to the U.S. Environmental Protection Agency, about twenty percent of all lung cancer cases in nonsmokers are thought to be related to secondhand smoke. A typical nonsmoker who lives with a smoker is unknowingly exposed to carcinogens equivalent to those found in up to twenty cigarettes per day. Babies are three times more likely to die at or shortly after birth if their mothers smoke during and after pregnancy.

We have all been brought up hearing that cigarette smoking causes lung cancer and that tobacco is a carcinogen. Few realize that all the cigarettes sold in North America are contaminated with fungi and have had sugar and yeast added to the final product. Sugar increases fungal growth. So does baker's or brewer's yeast. It is conceivable that tobacco itself is harmless and that it is commercially made carcinogenic partially due to fungal contamination. The mycotoxin *fusarium*, found in cigarettes, has been linked with lung cancer, esophageal cancer, and cancer of the uterus.

Protection from Cigarette Smoke

One of the best protections against the deleterious effects of tobacco smoke is the use of room air purifiers. Although there are many good types of air-filtering devices on the market, the HEPA (high-efficiency particulate accumulator) filter is the most widely accepted. It can remove all smoke and tars from the air as well as pollen, bacteria, and most viruses.

To help pull tar and nicotine out of the body, use Epsom salt baths (about half a pound of Epsom salts per bath).

Exercise, saunas, and bowel detoxification programs are also effective in ridding the body of toxins caused by cigarette smoke. Other forms of self-defense for nonsmokers exposed to second-hand smoke include the regular supplementation of the diet with the same antioxidant foods and nutrients that provide protection to smokers. These include the following foods and nutritional supplements:

Foods:

>   cooked beans (legumes)
>
>   eggs
>
>   garlic
>
>   onions

Green foods:

>   barley green
>
>   blue-green algae
>
>   chlorella
>
>   green kamut
>
>   liquid chlorophyll
>
>   spirulina

Vitamins, minerals, and other supplements:

>   B complex
>
>   beta carotene
>
>   choline
>
>   coenzyme Q10
>
>   colloidal silver

copper

cysteine

magnesium

methionine

selenium

silicon

vitamin A

vitamin C

vitamin E

zinc

Many companies market antioxidant supplements in a single pill or powder form for greater convenience.

Aspirin and Immunity

Practically every household in North America has aspirin in the medicine cabinet. Children commonly take it and often have their immune systems harmed as a result. Aspirin use in children has been associated with asthma, allergic rhinitis, kidney problems, inflammatory bowel disease, environmental hypersensitivities, liver problems, and bleeding disorders.

Potential side effects of aspirin:

- asthma, chronic rhinitis, and nasal polyps
- bleeding
- drowsiness
- excessive sweating and thirst
- gastrointestinal hemorrhage (ulcers)

- gastrointestinal irritation (heartburn, nausea, vomiting, diarrhea, inflammatory bowel disease)
- hearing loss
- hives (urticaria)
- hyperactivity
- increased gastric permeability and altered immunity
- inhibition of cartilage repair and accelerated cartilage destruction
- mental confusion
- Reye's syndrome
- ringing in the ears (tinnitus)
- vertigo

How Does Aspirin Work?

Aspirin prevents blood-clotting factors called platelets from sticking to each other. It does so by blocking a platelet enzyme called cyclooxygenase. By inhibiting the activity of cyclooxygenase, aspirin can decrease the production of lipid peroxides (free radicals) and thromboxane, a powerful vasoconstrictor. This enzyme inhibition lasts for the lifetime of the platelet, which is approximately ten days.

Aspirin also suppresses the activity of proinflammatory chemicals in the body known as the PGE2 family of prostaglandins. It thus indirectly increases the activity of anti-inflammatory prostaglandins of the PGE1 family. A natural substance called GLA (gamma linolenic acid), found in plants such as borage, black currant seed, and evening primrose, has also been shown to increase the activity of the PGE1 family, producing an anti-inflammatory effect similar to that of aspirin. Flaxseed oil (edible linseed oil) does not contain GLA but is rich in linoleic acid, which can be converted to GLA in the body to produce these same anti-inflammatory effects. GLA has been documented to lower serum cholesterol levels, reverse some cases of obesity, clear eczema, lower blood pressure, control allergies, counteract autoimmune disease, and prevent arthritis.

Natural Aspirin Alternatives

In addition to GLA, there are many safe and effective natural substances that can mimic the behavior of aspirin. It must be stressed, however, that if one consumes a lot of sugar, refined foods, and saturated fats (red meat, chicken, dairy products, etc.) and does not exercise, neither aspirin nor any of the following alternatives can be guaranteed to do much good.

Beta carotene: The best source of beta carotene is whole carrots. Equally good is a live whole-food concentrate of carrots. Eating carrots or swallowing live whole-food carrot concentrate capsules is therefore better than just drinking carrot juice, which in turn is better than just taking a beta carotene supplement. Carrot juice and carrots contain beta carotene, but they also contain small amounts of protein, carbohydrate, fat, fiber, potassium, vitamin C, and a long list of other essential nutrients.

Carrots and carrot juice are alkaline-forming foods. They lower the risk of cancer, especially smoking-related cancers such as lung cancer. One aspect of aspirin is its ability to protect against bowel cancer—beta carotene does the same. Carrots are excellent complementary treatments for all skin disorders and respiratory problems such as asthma and bronchitis. They may also be of help for gastrointestinal problems such as colitis, enteritis, and ulcers, probably because carotene and other carotenoids all help boost the immune system against bacterial, viral, fungal, and parasitic diseases as well as cancer.

Bioflavonoids: These are special antioxidant compounds found in green tea, grapes, vegetables such as peppers, and many fruits, especially berries and citrus. Some better-known bioflavonoids include catechin, hesperidin, rutin, quercetin, pycnogenol, pronogenol, and polyphenols. Bioflavonoids can lower LDL cholesterol levels and inhibit platelet stickiness much like aspirin. Together with vitamin C in large doses, bioflavonoids are also very effective in the treatment of allergies.

Devil's claw:　This herb originates in Africa and can be used as an alternative to prescription or nonprescription analgesics or anti-inflammatory agents in almost any situation. Devil's claw root (*harpagophytum procumbens*) has strong analgesic and anti-inflammatory properties. It has been documented to help with all types of arthritis and provides symptomatic relief of pain in neuralgia, headaches, heartburn, and constipation.

　　Devil's claw root contains many biochemically active compounds which function as free radical scavengers, while others have been shown to have anti-inflammatory properties. Like vitamin and mineral supplements, devil's claw root has a very low potential for side effects. In medically complicated cases, supervision by a health care practitioner is desirable.

Feverfew:　This safe, effective herb has benefits in the treatment of indigestion, sleeplessness, and headaches. It is another aspirin alternative and can be used safely in children.

Garlic:　A well-known herb, garlic prevents platelet stickiness and has natural antibacterial, antifungal, and antiparasitic properties.

Magnesium:　This mineral has anticoagulant properties which, when combined with vitamin E, can produce significant blood clotting reduction. It is always wise to balance magnesium intake with both calcium and potassium. Evaluation of blood and tissue levels can be done with the help of a health care practitioner.

Onions:　Onions retard platelet stickiness in much the same way as garlic.

Omega-3 EPA oils: These naturally help reduce inflammation and the symptoms of childhood allergies. They prevent platelet stickiness. Good dietary sources include flaxseed oil, rice bran oil, trout, mackerel, salmon, herring, sardines, cod, halibut, and shark.

Selenium: Selenium is an antioxidant which works in conjunction with vitamin E to protect vascular tissue from damage by toxins. It is also strongly antifungal.

Vitamin B-6:   Vitamin B-6 has blood clotting retarding effects and is best taken in the form of a B complex vitamin supplement to fully balance all the B vitamins.

Vitamin C: This vitamin has anti-inflammatory effects as well as antihistamine effects.

Vitamin E: This is otherwise known as alpha-tocopherol. High doses have been shown to retard blood clotting. Caution should be exercised if one is using both aspirin and vitamin E because the combination has a synergistic effect.

High-dose vitamin E supplements can interfere with iron absorption, so iron supplements should be taken about twelve hours apart from vitamin E supplements.

White willow bark (Salix alba):   This contains salicin, from which aspirin is manufactured. While not as potent as aspirin, white willow has very similar properties at therapeutic dosages without significant side effects. White willow has anti-inflammatory, antipyretic, analgesic, antiseptic, and astringent properties, with far fewer gastrointestinal side effects than aspirin. It has a wide variety of uses for the symptomatic relief or control of pain, connective tissue inflammation, headaches, muscle aches, fevers, chronic diarrhea, and dysentery.

Massive doses of white willow can produce toxicity similar to that seen with aspirin, but this is extremely rare. White willow contains salicin and tannins and prevents platelet stickiness. It is not recommended for use before surgery. A health practitioner's supervision is recommended whenever dosages prescribed are higher than those recommended on the label.

Yucca: Due to its high content of saponins, this herb has antiinflammatory as well as blood-purifying properties. It has no side effects and works synergistically with licorice root, alfalfa, devil's claw, and white willow.

Many of these nutrients are sold in combination form at health food stores. A naturopath or medical doctor familiar with these remedies can recommend specific dosages. Discuss all the options with your health care practitioner, and use his or her experience and expertise to guide you with an individualized health program.

The Vaccination Controversy

One of the most common questions asked of me by parents at my office is whether they should vaccinate their children. This is not a cut-and-dried decision.

Vaccinations are regarded as an essential part of modern medicine, and its practice is enforced by various government agencies.

But over the past decade, many scientists from around the world have pointed out the lack of credible studies proving that repeated use of multiple vaccines is safe and effective as advertised. There is also some evidence that vaccines cause immune and neurological dysfunction in childhood and later life.

The persecution of physicians such as Dr. Guylaine Lanctot, who has publicized the risks of vaccination, continues to fuel the vaccine controversy because the persecutors are unable to present evidence or justification for their actions.

Vaccines are the only product sold in North America that carry the risk of injury or death and which are legally required to be used by every healthy citizen. Until the late 1980s, few questioned the wisdom of this requirement. However, a growing segment of the population, including many in the alternative health care community, question the wisdom of injecting foreign proteins, aluminum, mercury derivatives, formaldehyde, unknown genetic material, and possible contaminants into a child's bloodstream. They worry about the growing number of reports on the association between vaccines and hyperactivity, autism, seizure disorders, chronic ear infections, hearing impairment, diabetes, allergies, asthma, mental retardation, and autoimmune diseases.

On the other hand, well respected doctors, pediatricians, and medical journals say that vaccines are safe and effective. Campaigns originating from respected organizations—the government, medical groups, and school committees—and the repeated message in the news media declare the importance of vaccination. No wonder many parents are confused. The information presented here is intended to help parents sort out fact from fiction and make informed decisions about vaccinating their children. After seeing the damage caused by mass vaccinations in my own practice, I am not completely convinced of either their safety or efficacy.

Some Evidence Against Vaccination

> If I could live my life over again, I would devote it to proving that germs seek their natural habitat—diseased tissue—rather than being the cause of the "diseased" tissue.
>
> —*Rudolph Virchow, M.D.*

A large number of reputable scientists point out that the germ theory of disease has never been adequately proven. Some studies conclude that up to ninety percent of the decrease in infectious disease occurred before the introduction of vaccines or antibiotics. As an example, scarlet fever has disappeared despite the fact that there has never been a vaccine or treatment for it.

My experience, both as a physician and as a past president of a medical organization, is that the mainstream health communities selectively publicize only what they want us to know about vaccines. My intention here is to give you the other side of the story.

Vaccinations can have negative consequences:

• Within a thirty-nine-month period ending November 1993, the Food and Drug Administration's Vaccine Adverse Events Reporting System collected nearly 32,000 reports of adverse reactions following vaccination, with more than 700 deaths. DPT (diphtheria, pertussis, tetanus) vaccine was associated with more than 12,000 of these reports, including 471 deaths. This was voluntary reporting which even the FDA acknowledges underestimated the actual number of reactions and deaths. These reports of illness and deaths are dismissed by most doctors and government officials as "statistically insignificant."

• Five to fifteen percent of children receiving the measles vaccine react with a mild rash or fever. Some research also indicates that the measles vaccine can be responsible for meningitis, seizure disorders, mental retardation, and muscle abnormalities.

• Side effects of the MMR (measles, mumps, rubella) and polio vaccinations include anaphylactic shock, arthritis, conjunctivitis, cough and/or coryza, fever, general rashes (acute hives), Guillain-Barre syndrome, irritability, local erythemas (redness), multiple sclerosis, peripheral tremor, post-vaccinal meningitis (aseptic meningitis), and tiredness.

• Immunizations can lead to a deterioration from existing autoimmune diseases. According to many experts, it is usually advisable for those suffering from such conditions not to get further vaccinations.

- Many authors suspect an association between vaccinations and conditions such as AIDS, SIDS (sudden infant death syndrome), encephalitis, multiple sclerosis, rheumatoid arthritis, Lou Gehrig's disease, Guillain-Barre syndrome, lupus, and leukemia.

- The British National Childhood Encephalopathy Study (NCES), conducted in 1988, concluded that there was a relationship between neurological illness and diphtheria-pertussis-tetanus (DPT) immunization in children two to thirty-six months of age.

- According to Dr. Harris Coulter, author of two books analyzing the impact of mass vaccinations, the incidence of epilepsy and seizure disorders increased in 1945, at around the same time that the United States started its mass vaccination program. A study of 500,000 children by the Centers for Disease Control and Prevention in Atlanta reported that the seizure rate among children given the MMR shot rose 2.7 times within four to seven days, and increased to 3.3 times within fourteen days (article by Clive Couldwell appeared in *What Doctors Don't Tell You*, vol. 6, no. 8, Dec. 1995).

- The 1994 measles campaign in Great Britain discovered that the mumps element in the MMR vaccine caused meningitis in at least one in eleven thousand cases. In one area of Japan, the incidence of meningitis was one in five hundred children vaccinated with the MMR injection.

Vaccines often don't work: The Centers for Disease Control (CDC) in the United States reported that, in the first half of 1987, over half of the reported measles cases were in children who had been fully vaccinated. The Ohio Department of Health (ODH) reported that 2,720 children developed measles in 1989 despite the fact that close to three-fourths of the cases occurred in previously vaccinated children. In a 1984 CDC report in *Morbidity and Mortality Weekly Report,* measles outbreaks were reported in a population documented as being one hundred percent vaccinated.

The CDC reported the following in a 1989 issue of *Morbidity and Mortality Weekly Reports:*

> Among school-aged children, [measles] outbreaks have occurred in schools with vaccination levels of greater than ninety-eight percent. These outbreaks have occurred in all parts of the country, including areas that had not reported measles for years.

Half of the reported pertussis (whooping cough) cases in Ohio between 1987 and 1991 occurred in children who were vaccinated. One 1989 study in the *Journal of Pediatrics* reported a fifty-five-percent failure rate for the pertussis vaccine.

In late 1993, Cincinnati, St. Louis, Chicago, and Philadelphia experienced highly publicized pertussis epidemics. A July 7, 1994, *New England Journal of Medicine* article reported that the 352 pertussis cases in Cincinnati occurred primarily among children who had been appropriately immunized. Similarly, of 186 confirmed pertussis cases in Chicago, the Chicago Department of Health noted, "Seventy-two percent were as up-to-date as possible on their immunizations for their age."

The mumps vaccine is also highly ineffective, with outbreaks often occurring in vaccinated preschool and school-age children, according to a 1989 *Journal of Pediatrics* article. A large-scale mumps epidemic outbreak occurred in April 1993 in a vaccinated population in Nashville, Tennessee. Studies show that the immunization against mumps provides only seventy-five percent protection.

Other esteemed studies indicate that vaccinated children contract the very diseases against which they were vaccinated at the same or higher rates than unvaccinated children. The claim that the diseases that vaccinated children do develop are milder is unproven. On the contrary, there is mounting evidence that measles in vaccinated children can be much more serious than in unvaccinated kids.

Revaccination also doesn't work. Because the first MMR vaccine was found to be ineffective, the CDC and the American Academy of Pediatrics recommended a second dose of the MMR vaccine just before kindergarten, seventh grade, or college.

Even ideal vaccines may not be necessary: Dr. Robert Mendelsohn, Dr. Leon Chaitow, and others claim that better nutrition and living conditions, such as improved sanitation, are probably the cause of the reductions in childhood diseases rather than vaccinations.

Furthermore, traditional Chinese medical practitioners believe that measles, mumps, and chicken pox are beneficial childhood diseases that boost immunity and help rid the body of harmful poisons.

According to a 1990 publication by 180 Swiss doctors who make up the Medical Working Group, no one has ever published a double-blind study to determine if a measles vaccine is significantly better than a neutral placebo.

The Medical Working Group believes that childhood illnesses are important to the maturation and development of the immune system in defending itself against allergies, infections, asthma, eczema, and even cancer. Suppressing normal childhood illnesses could well backfire on the population as a whole.

For example, the prevalence of parasites and the average density of malaria parasites are significantly lower in children who have had measles or influenza before the age of nine than in an asymptomatic control group. Persons who have never had any visible indication of measles suffer more frequently from autoimmune diseases, seborrheic skin diseases, degenerative diseases of the bones, and certain tumors.

The theory about why this happens has to do with how the immune system responds to an invader. If the infection with measles happens at a time when there are already antibodies against the measles virus present, i.e., within the first few months after birth in the measles-immunized child, the immune system cannot react fully to the infection, giving the virus the chance to become persistent, later developing into an autoimmune disease and other chronic allergic problems. This theory remains to be proven.

Along similar lines, several authors have postulated a cross-reaction between foreign pathogens (or vaccines) and the body's own tissues in the development of conditions such as juvenile rheumatoid arthritis. If one introduces a foreign substance (a vaccine) into the body, which has a similar structure as some body tissue, the production of antibodies against that foreign substance could also lead these antibodies to attack that body tissue (an autoimmune reaction).

Vaccination and the Development of Childhood Allergies

Neurodermatitis, hay fever, asthma, the hyperkinetic syndrome, eczema, chronic fatigue syndrome, fibromyalgia, multiple sclerosis, and psoriasis have all been associated with food and chemical allergies. Many pediatricians blame the rising incidence of these allergic conditions on too-early ingestion of commonly allergenic foods. The early introduction of allergens into a child's diet, or given as an injection, has been documented to increase the incidence of chronic allergic illness. For example, a study of more than two thousand children showed that feeding them cow's milk during the first nine months resulted in seven times more frequent complaints of eczema afterward.

Despite such reports, children are aggressively exposed to foreign proteins (allergens) at a very early age in the form of immunizations (diphtheria, tetanus, pertussis, poliomyelitis, Haemophilus influenzae, measles, mumps, rubella, and all the corresponding booster shots). Vaccines contain carcinogenic toxins (formaldehyde and Thimerosal) and are being injected into two-, four-, and six-month-old infants whose immune systems are not fully developed.

The fact that doctors, on the one hand, advise parents to avoid early childhood contact with allergens such as cow's milk and eggs while, on the other hand, massively promoting it by means of vaccinations seems illogical. Given the growing severity of immune diseases in children, especially asthma, shouldn't there first be studies on the connection between immunizations and subsequent immune system impairment? If conventional medical authorities demand proof of the safety and efficacy of natural remedies before they are to be recommended to children, why isn't the same proof demanded for vaccinations?

How Parents Can Legally Refuse Vaccinations

> Who then can so softly bind up the wound of another as he who has felt the same wound himself?
>
> —*Thomas Jefferson*

Despite what they may have been led to believe, parents do have a choice about vaccinating their children. Every state has a medical exemption, forty-eight states have a religious exemption, and sixteen states have a philosophical exemption available for parents who choose not to vaccinate their children. Although poorly publicized, all Canadian provinces allow exemptions for medical or religious reasons.

Legally, you are entitled to say "no" to any vaccine. Confronting worried relatives, schools, doctors, and medical officials is difficult at best. My advice to those who wish to say "no" is to contact the groups listed in Appendix IV to find out what the laws are in your location. These groups can also provide you with a great deal of information to help you make an informed decision about vaccinating your children.

6   Creating Childhood Superimmunity

All truth goes through three stages. First it is ridiculed. Then it is violently opposed. Finally, it is accepted as self-evident.

—*Arthur Schopenhauer*

The best way to keep children healthy is to create a state of superimmunity in their bodies, whereby there is an optimal state of health as opposed to simply a normal one. By taking a proactive approach to health and prevention through nutritional, environmental, and lifestyle changes, optimal health can be achieved for children.

Superimmune children are:

- vibrant in appearance, with high energy levels
- above average in their resistance to disease
- free of allergies, autoimmune disease, and degenerative disease
- above average in mental functioning and emotional maturity

Step One: Antioxidants

Free radicals are highly reactive molecules that bind to and destroy cells, tissues, and organs in the body through oxidation reactions. Recent well-publicized research concludes that free radicals originating from digestion by-products, food, water, air pollution, radiation, cigarettes, alcohol, and drugs are responsible for aging and the initiation of heart disease, cancer, and other degenerative diseases, even in children.

Most brands of cigarettes, soda, processed cheese, processed soup, beer, laundry detergent, and coffee contain chemicals that have been proven to cause free radical damage. Despite increased education in the areas of nutrition and lifestyle, the majority of North American children continue to be exposed to a daily onslaught of free radicals coming from cigarettes, processed foods, cleaning products, caffeine, and numerous drugs. They get too little exercise, watch too much television, and eat a diet high in fat and low in fiber. And at least thirty percent of North Americans smoke cigarettes and pass on their unhealthy habits to their children.

The body attempts to protect itself from free radical damage through antioxidant nutrients such as selenium, zinc, beta carotene, vitamin E, glutathione, vitamin C, and bioflavonoids such as grape-seed extract (proanthocyaniclins), rutin, hesperidin, quercetin, and catechin. Unfortunately, the overall poor nutrition and lifestyle habits of North Americans deplete the body of its reserves of antioxidants.

Over two hundred published scientific and peer-reviewed studies indicate that supplementation of antioxidants (free radical quenchers) is effective preventive medicine against allergies, cancer, heart disease, cataracts, diabetes, arthritis, recurrent infections, all skin diseases, and chronic immune system disorders. Given the worsening quality of our environment, antioxidant supplementation may be one of the only practical defenses against free radical damage. The typical urban food supply or multivitamin will not provide adequate antioxidant protection. For these and other reasons, daily antioxidant supplements are essential for children to become superimmune.

Step Two: Natural Interferon Boosters

Interferon is produced naturally by the body's white cells to fight and prevent viral and other infections, cancer, allergies, and chemical toxic poisoning of the body. A fever stimulates the body to make more interferon, one of the reasons why naturo-paths recommend against the use of drugs to suppress fevers. Interferon can stimulate the immune system to produce more of the disease-fighting T-cells. These are the white blood cells which combat viruses, bacteria, and other microbes.

Many natural substances have been shown to stimulate the body's natural production of interferon. Some of the best-known and documented ones are listed below.

Astragalus: A well-known Chinese herb that enhances the anti-body reaction to antigens occuring in allergies, infection, and cancer. It increases T-lymphocyte activity, improves clinical signs and symptoms of many HIV-related problems, and increases the body's production of interferon.

Beta carotene: May act to prevent the development of allergies and other childhood illnesses through its interferon-stimulating ability as well as its antioxidant properties. Beta carotene is not toxic to the liver even in high doses. Large doses of beta carotene increase the body's demands for vitamin E, so if one takes 50,000 to 100,000 units of beta carotene per day, vitamin E intake should be increased to 1,000 to 2,000 units per day. Beta carotene, like vitamins A and E, is stored in the liver.

Boneset: An herb used successfully by Native Americans for the treatment of colds and flu, coughs, fevers, indigestion, and pain. It has antiseptic properties, promotes sweating, is antiviral, and boosts the immune system by enhancing the body's own secre-tion of interferon.

Chlorophyll: Can be found in a long list of green leafy vegeta-bles and green products such as spirulina, chlorella, blue-green algae, barley green, and dozens of others. One of the best rea-sons for eating greens is for their chlorophyll content.

Coenzyme Q10 (coQ10):   An accessory food factor involved in the electron transport chain, a system which is important for all energy-dependent processes in the body. CoQ10 boosts interferon production, increases the level of helper T-cells, and reduces the risk for opportunistic infections. Periodontal disease responds very well to high doses of coQ10.

Comfrey: An herb that stimulates not only interferon production but also T-cell and B-cell activity and macrophage phagocytosis. T-cells and B-cells are the white cells which manufacture antibodies against foreign invaders. A macrophage is a type of white blood cell that pursues and engulfs germs in the blood through the process of phagocytosis.

Comfrey has been used for centuries for the healing of wounds, strains, sprains, and fractures and for bone repair and bone strengthening. Comfrey encourages strong bones and healthy skin by helping the calcium-phosphorus balance. It also promotes the secretion of pepsin and is an aid to good digestion. It is often used for overall health enhancement and to treat asthma, arthritis, and ulcers.

Dong quai: An herb used by the Chinese for at least two thousand years as a tonic for all female problems. Research has proven that dong quai has antitumor, antifungal, antibacterial, and immune-stimulating properties. It stimulates the production of interferon and increases circulation by helping to dissolve blood clots.

Echinacea: An herb used by North American Indians as a treatment for toothaches, snake bites, insect bites or stings, and all types of infections. It has a reputation as a blood purifier and is found to have interferon-like properties. It fights strep, staph, and candida (yeast) infections and can kill fungi. It has been used successfully to treat blood poisoning, ulcers, tuberculosis, childhood infections of every kind, and a long list of skin, digestive, and immune system disorders. Most herbalists recommend that echinacea be used on an intermittent basis: three weeks on, two weeks off, and so on, because its immune-boosting effects fail to occur if used continuously. In very high dosages (taken every hour or more often), echinacea is effective as a pain control remedy. In coughs, sore throats, and other irritations, it is best consumed as a tincture. Echinacea increases the ability of the body to resist infections, removes toxins from the blood, and improves lymphatic filtration and drainage.

Germanium: A trace mineral, the organic form of which is used by many practitioners for the treatment of chronic fatigue, allergies, infections, and cancer. Part of its efficacy comes from its ability to boost interferon. A good source of naturally occurring germanium is Korean ginseng.

Ginkgo: A potent central nervous system antioxidant useful in the treatment of circulation problems, memory problems, high blood pressure, depression, tinnitus, and immune system disorders through its ability to boost interferon levels. It can help children improve learning and memory.

Ho-shou-wu: An herb highly regarded by the Chinese for treating liver, spleen, and heart problems. It can help reduce cholesterol levels and inflammation. *Ho-shou-wu* strengthens the heart, has antiviral properties via enhanced interferon production, and has calming effects on the nervous system.

Licorice: Has been used by many cultures worldwide as a tonic, and a treatment for infections, digestive problems, ulcers, hepatitis, Addison's disease, adrenal insufficiency, and congestion. Licorice has anti-inflammatory and antiallergic properties. The two components of licorice—glycyrrhizin and glycyrrhetinic acid—stimulate the production of interferon by the body. Licorice is very helpful in treating coughs, colds, and the flu and heals inflamed mucous membranes in the respiratory tract. It increases the number of antibodies, activates the production of interferon, and slows the growth of tumors. It can be taken as a tea, tincture, or capsule. In large doses, some sensitive individuals develop high blood pressure from licorice. For this reason, long-term use of licorice should be supervised by a naturopath or holistic medical doctor.

Marshmallow herb: Stimulates not only interferon production but also T-cell and B-cell activity and macrophage phagocytosis. It is soothing to the mucous membranes and acts as an anti-inflammatory.

Medicinal mushrooms: Reishi, maitake, shiitake, Kombucha, and others stimulate many aspects of the immune system, including the production of interferon. The *maitake* mushroom (*Grifola frondosa*) has been prized in Japanese herbalogy for hundreds of years to strengthen the body and improve overall health. Studies indicate that compounds (beta glucan) contained in *maitake* can stimulate immune function and inhibit tumor growth. *Maitake* mushroom benefits people with HIV/AIDS because it can prevent the destruction of helper T-cells by the virus. Many other conditions including diabetes and obesity respond very well to *maitake* treatment.

Melatonin: A hormone produced by the pineal gland which has strong antioxidant properties and has been shown to act on the immune system by causing the release of cytokines from activated T-cell populations. Melatonin increases the production of interferon but has become popular for a variety of other reasons. Melatonin has been gaining a reputation for being able to prevent many diseases, especially cancer. Most antioxidant nutrients have difficulty penetrating cell membranes, while melatonin does not. Several scientists believe that melatonin may prove to be the most important free radical scavenger yet discovered.

Some of the many childhood diseases thought to be alleviated by melatonin are muscular dystrophy, rheumatoid arthritis, and epilepsy. New studies indicate that melatonin may have a restorative effect on thymic function by inducing the optimal growth and functioning of the gland, increasing production of T-cells, and increasing secretion of the thymus hormones, thymosin and thymulin. There is no evidence that it can be harmful to children, but dosages should start at very low levels and be slowly increased under the supervision of a natural health care practitioner.

Milk thistle (silymarin):   An herbal remedy most commonly used as a liver cleanser and as complementary medical treatment for hepatitis and liver congestion. It also has interferon-stimulating effects in the body.

Pau d'arco (taheebo):   Well-known for its antifungal effects as well as its immune-system-stimulating properties. Several anecdotal reports have indicated that *pau d'arco* could have cancer-reversing properties through its ability to boost interferon levels.

Plantago (psyllium seed):   Known by many names, including pharmacy brands. It stimulates not only interferon production but also T-cell and B-cell activity and macrophage phagocytosis (see section about comfrey root). Current FDA (HPB in Canada) regulations prevent any claims for cancer and infection prevention for any commercial products containing psyllium.

Red raspberry: Has antiviral properties due to its ability to stimulate the production of interferon and is a healthy addition to any child's regime of herbal supplements.

Schizandra: A popular Chinese herb that has antibacterial and antiviral properties via its interferon effects. It protects the liver from toxins, boosts stamina, and protects the body from free radical damage.

Sea vegetables: Kelp, dulse, blue-green algae, chlorella, and spirulina are just some of the better-known sea plants capable of boosting interferon levels.

Siberian ginseng: Stimulates not only interferon production but also T-cell and B-cell activity and macrophage phagocytosis. In addition, it has energy-boosting properties, helps burn off extra fat through its thermogenic effects, and improves mental functioning, IQ, and circulation.

Suma: An herb originating in the rain forests of Brazil and used as a tonic, energy booster, and antidiabetic remedy. It has antiviral and anticancer properties, partly due to its ability to increase interferon levels.

Vitamin C and bioflavonoids: Antioxidants that help in treatment of a cold, cough, or flu. A high vitamin C intake stimulates the production of hydrogen peroxide. In the blood, our white blood cells (lymphocytes) produce hydrogen peroxide to combat invasive organisms. The only significant side effects of taking vitamin C are diarrhea and flatulence. Dosages should be reduced if the side effects become too uncomfortable.

Vitamin C is an interferon booster. It also promotes healthy cell development, improved wound healing, and resistance to infections. It may help protect against allergies, autoimmune diseases, and asthma. Vitamin C will help with the healing of burns. It improves the strength of the walls of the blood vessels and may help decrease easy bruising. Vitamin C may help people with low back pain and arthritis due to its antioxidant effects.

Bioflavonoids are vital in their ability to increase the strength of the capillaries and to regulate their permeability. They assist vitamin C in maintaining levels of collagen, the intercellular "cement," in healthy condition. Bioflavonoids are essential for the proper absorption and use of vitamin C and for preventing vitamin C from being destroyed in the body by oxidation. Bioflavonoids prevent hemorrhages, excessive menstrual bleeding, and ruptures in the capillaries and connective tissues.

Bioflavonoids can be ingested through grape-seed extract, pine-bark extract, and bilberry.

Wheat grass: An interferon booster used as a juice. Many alternative medical centers use it as a cancer-fighting agent.

Step Three: Other Supplements

The following supplements are to be used in cases of deficiency, increased risk for certain diseases, or as dictated by special circumstances. These are all best taken under the supervision by a qualified health care practitioner.

Biotin: A water-soluble B vitamin that acts as a coenzyme in the production of fatty acids and in the oxidation of fatty acids and carbohydrates. Biotin in high dosages is antifungal and has been found to be effective therapeutically in treating seborrheic dermatitis ("cradle cap" in children), uremia in patients on dialysis, diabetes (may be helpful for peripheral neuropathy), dermatitis, and muscle pains. It is depleted by antibiotics, sulfa drugs, and the avidin found in eggs. It has no known toxicity.

Calcium: Builds and maintains bones and teeth, regulates heart rhythm, eases insomnia, helps regulate the passage of nutrients in and out of the cell walls, assists in normal blood clotting, helps maintain proper nerve and muscle function, lowers blood pressure, and is important to normal kidney function. Calcium deficiency may result in arm and leg muscle spasms, softening of bones, back and leg cramps, brittle bones, rickets, poor growth, osteoporosis, tooth decay, and depression. (See Chapter 3 for more information on sources of calcium.)

Choline: One of the B complex vitamins, it functions with inositol as a basic constituent of lecithin. Choline is part of the cell membrane structure, transports fat-soluble substances, is important in nerve impulse transmission, and may help the brain to reason, learn, and remember. Choline is effective therapeutically in headaches, liver damage, hepatitis, and learning disorders. Sugar and many drugs deplete choline. Prolonged megadoses of choline may induce a vitamin B-6 deficiency; it is therefore recommended to take choline as part of the B complex vitamins.

Copper: A mineral necessary for the absorption and utilization of iron. It works with vitamin C to form elastin, a chief component of the elastin muscle fibers throughout the body. Copper aids in the formation of red blood cells and helps proper bone formation and maintenance. Copper deficiency may result in general weakness, impaired respiration, skin sores, and joint pains.

Broken bones heal faster when children are given copper during the period of convalescence. Copper is necessary in the biosynthesis of bone and connective tissues. Inadequate copper intake leads to improper bone formation and bone fractures in newborns, infants, young children, and sometimes even adults. This is because several enzymes, such as lysyl oxidase, which mediate the synthesis of collagen are copper-dependent enzymes. Other copper-dependent enzymes include ceruloplasmin, cytochrome oxidase, and superoxide dismutase, all of which play vital roles in protecting the body against injuries and free radical damage. Severe copper deficiency can cause brain damage, impaired growth, retinal dystrophy, arterial disease, osteoporosis, and sudden death due to rupture of the heart or a major artery (aneurysm).

While copper is important for health and wound healing, it is potentially harmful if its intake is excessive. Copper, like iron, is a trace metal that should be ingested solely through the diet, unless there is a clear-cut copper deficiency. Good dietary sources of copper include beans, peas, green leafy vegetables, prunes, raisins, liver, seafood, lamb, and soybeans.

Dahlia inulin: A relatively new natural food supplement that can be useful in children who have weight-control problems, low energy, blood sugar control problems, a craving for sweets, or recurrent infections. Dahlia inulin is a complex carbohydrate that controls abnormal appetite behavior. It basically prevents hunger caused by excessively low blood sugar levels. After intake, it can help stabilize blood sugar levels for up to ten hours. It provides a good growth medium for the friendly bacterial flora known as bifidobacteria, which are important in the prevention of infectious diseases. Inulin minimizes the breakdown of muscle tissue during exercise and increases total energy reserves.

Essential fatty acids (EFAs): Must be obtained from the diet or supplements because the body cannot make EFAs from other substances. Children are especially vulnerable to the signs and symptoms of essential fatty acid deficiency due to lowfat diets.

Two fatty acids are essential to human health:

1. Omega-6 EFA (linoleic acid [LA] family), which is abundant in polyunsaturated safflower, sunflower, and corn oils. The LA family includes gamma-linoleic acid (GLA), dihomogamma-linolenic acid (DGLA), and arachidonic acid (AA).
2. Omega-3 EFA (alpha-linolenic acid [ALA] family), which is found abundantly in flaxseed and hemp seeds. The omega-3 family includes eicosapentaenoic acid (EPA) and docosahexaenoic acid (DHA).

Our cells make GLA, DGLA, and AA from essential fatty acid precursors. A high intake of unhealthy fats such as margarine, shortening, trans-fatty acids, hard fats, and cholesterol can inhibit this omega-6 conversion. So can a high sugar intake. A lack of magnesium, selenium, zinc, and vitamins B-3, B-6, C, and E can also inhibit this conversion. So can viruses (as can occur in chronic fatigue syndrome), obesity, diabetes, and rare genetic mutations. In all these cases, supplementation present in evening primrose, borage, and black currant seed can help.

DGLA is found in mother's milk, while AA is found in meats, eggs, and dairy products. When the conversion of EFAs to their derivatives is inhibited by the same factors which inhibit omega-6 conversion, DHA from black currant seed oil, or EPA and DHA from fish oils and northern ocean algae, can be given.

Essential fatty acids:

• Help form the membrane barrier that surrounds our cells and intracellular structures (organelles)

- Determine the fluidity and chemical reactivity of membranes
- Increase oxidation rate, metabolic rate, and energy levels
- Serve as starting material for prostaglandins—hormones that have a strong influence on inflammation, pain, and allergic response
- Carry oil-soluble toxins from deep within the body to the skin surface for elimination
- Store electric charges that produce bioelectric currents important for nerve, muscle, and cell membrane functions and the transmission of messages
- Help form a barrier that keeps foreign molecules, viruses, yeasts, fungi, and bacteria outside of cells and keeps the cell's proteins, enzymes, genetic material, and organelles inside
- Help regulate the traffic of substances in and out of our cells via protein channels, pumps, and other mechanisms
- Regulate oxygen use, electron transport, and energy production
- Help form red blood pigment (hemoglobin)
- Keep juice-producing (exocrine) and hormone-producing (endocrine) glands active
- Help make joint lubricants
- Are precursors of prostaglandins (PGs)—hormones that regulate blood pressure, platelet stickiness, and kidney function
- Determine the health of our cardiovascular system
- Help transport cholesterol; supplementation may help lower high cholesterol levels
- Help generate electrical currents that make our heart beat in an orderly sequence
- Are precursors of derivatives such as DHA, which are needed by the most active tissues: brain, retina, adrenal gland, and testes

- Help our immune system fight infections by enhancing peroxide (a naturally produced antibiotic) production

- Help prevent the development of allergies

Folic acid: A water-soluble vitamin which acts as a coenzyme in the conversion of glucose to energy.

Inositol: Part of the vitamin B complex and associated with choline and biotin. Inositol aids in the metabolism of fats and controls blood cholesterol. It is required as a nutrient for the cells of the brain, bone marrow, eye membranes, and the intestine. Inositol is important as part of the natural treatment of diabetes, alopecia, constipation, insomnia, hypercholesterolemia, hypertension, and schizophrenia. It is depleted or antagonized by antibiotics and has no known toxicity.

L-arginine: An amino acid (building block of proteins) that is essential during periods of stress in children, such as infections and traumatic physical injury. Following injury, there is a significantly increased need for L-arginine for a variety of metabolic functions. L-arginine speeds wound healing by increasing the pancreatic synthesis of insulin and glucagon, increasing the pituitary gland's synthesis of growth hormone and prolactin, increasing the size of the thymus gland and improving its function, and improving a variety of immune system functions, such as the activation of cells (macrophages) involved in tissue repair.

     L-arginine is probably best known for its ability to increase growth hormone release. Growth hormone plays a critical role in modulating the action of the immune system and is essential for muscle growth and development. Being underweight or undersized and having weakly developed muscles are some of the common childhood problems which may be helped by L-arginine supplementation.

Magnesium: Plays an important role in regulating the neuro-muscular activity of the heart. Magnesium has been referred to as "nature's calcium channel blocker." Calcium channel blockers prevent the influx and deposit of calcium in the arteries and soft tissues. Magnesium maintains normal heart rhythm, is necessary for proper calcium and vitamin C metabolism, and converts blood sugar into energy. Low magnesium levels may result in calcium depletion, heart spasms, nervousness, muscular excitability, confusion, chronic fatigue, and constipation.

Manganese: An antioxidant nutrient important in the blood breakdown of amino acids and insulin. It is therefore important in the production of energy, carbohydrate tolerance, and the metabolism of vitamin B-1 and vitamin E. Manganese activates various enzymes that are important for proper digestion and utilization of foods, is a catalyst in the breakdown of fats and cholesterol, and helps nourish the nerves and brain. Manganese is necessary for normal skeletal development. Deficiency may result in paralysis, convulsions, dizziness, ataxia, loss of hearing, digestive problems, blindness, and deafness in infants. Manganese, along with zinc and copper, stimulates the antioxidant enzyme SOD (superoxide dismutase). SOD is believed to be the mechanism by which these three minerals produce their analgesic and anti-inflammatory effects in different types of arthritis.

Selenium: A trace element that's been shown to be a very potent anticarcinogen, antioxidant, and natural anti-inflammatory agent. It is used as an effective remedy in rheumatoid arthritis, various muscular wasting diseases such as myotonic dystrophy, and lung diseases such as cystic fibrosis, all of which occur more frequently in children with selenium deficiencies. Studies indicate that selenium supplementation can prevent hepatitis and immunodeficiency diseases.

Selenium is one of the nutrients that can increase body levels of glutathione. Glutathione and its related compounds protect our cells from outside invaders and neutralize excessive free radical reactions within cells, especially those produced by the mitochondria.

Vitamin B-1 (thiamin): A water-soluble vitamin that acts as a coenzyme in the conversion of glucose to energy and helps the nervous system function normally. It is important in the treatment of beriberi, multiple sclerosis, myasthenia gravis, depression, anxiety, trigeminal neuralgia, and anemia. It is antagonized by alcohol, antibiotics, diuretics, and sugar. Thiamin has no known toxicity, but large doses may cause B complex imbalances.

Vitamin B-2 (riboflavin 5 phosphate): A water-soluble vitamin necessary for cell respiration, the production and utilization of energy in the body cells, and the promotion of healthy skin and eyes. It is useful in the treatment of visual disturbances, depression, acne rosacea, anemia, and eczema. It is antagonized by alcohol and antibiotics. It has no known toxicity, but large doses may result in increased urinary excretion of other B vitamins, leading to imbalances.

Vitamin B-3 (niacinamide): A water-soluble vitamin which has three synthetic forms: niacinamide, nicotinic acid, and nicotinamide. Niacinamide is the version of B-3 that does not cause the skin to turn red (nicotinic acid and niacin can cause a severe red flush on the skin). It aids fat metabolism, tissue respiration, and carbohydrate utilization. It promotes healthy skin, nerves, and digestion. Niacinamide can act as an effective natural tranquilizer for children because it affects the same receptors in the brain as the commonly prescribed tranquilizers called benzodiazepines.

Vitamin B-3 is often prescribed for blood sugar control problems, atherosclerosis, schizophrenia, hyperactivity, anxiety, multiple sclerosis, Bell's palsy, trigeminal neuralgia, tardive dyskinesia, diabetic neuropathy, dysmenorrhea, osteoarthritis, and fatigue. In megadoses, it may aggravate gout, put stress on the liver, and elevate blood sugar levels. Niacinamide is antagonized by alcohol, sugar, and antibiotics.

Vitamin B-5 (pantothenic acid): A water-soluble part of the vitamin B complex that stimulates the adrenal cortex, it is involved in the synthesis of cholesterol, steroids, and fatty acids, is a coenzyme in cellular metabolism, and maintains a healthy gastrointestinal tract. It has been used therapeutically for hypoglycemia, constipation, adrenal exhaustion, insomnia, epilepsy, multiple sclerosis, neuritis, fainting spells, depression, stress, cataracts, asthma, gastritis, indigestion, nausea, duodenal ulcers, arthritis, contact dermatitis, eczema, psoriasis, acne, and anemia. It is antagonized by aspirin and methylbromide. It has no known toxicity.

Vitamin B-6 (pyridoxine): A water-soluble vitamin consisting of three related compounds: pyridoxine, pyridoxal, and pyridoxamine. Vitamin B-6 assists in red blood cell regeneration, helps regulate protein, fat, and carbohydrate use, and is needed as a cofactor for neurotransmitters (dopamine, serotonin, norepinephrine, GABA). B-6 is used therapeutically for carpal tunnel syndrome, infant seizures, rheumatism, tardive dyskinesia, depression, dementia, hyperactivity, schizophrenia, seborrheic dermatitis, acne, anemia, atherosclerosis, asthma, monosodium glutamate sensitivity, kidney stones, and diabetes. Vitamin B-6 is antagonized by prescription hormones such as cortisone and estrogens used in various childhood metabolic disorders. Large doses may result in increased urinary excretion of other B vitamins, leading to imbalances and symptoms resembling mild paralysis (neuropathy).

Vitamin B-12 (hydroxycobalamin): A water-soluble vitamin that aids in the maintenance of nerve tissues and normal blood formation. It is a cofactor in transferring methyl groups and is effective therapeutically in pernicious anemia and for treating immune problems such as allergies, canker sores, viral hepatitis, herpes zoster, asthma, diabetic neuropathy, neuralgias, fatigue, bursitis, metatarsalgia, and skin problems such as psoriasis, seborrheic dermatitis, and eczema. It has no known toxicity.

Vitamin E: Otherwise known as alpha-tocopherol. Vitamin E acts as a free radical scavenger to keep the by-products of cell metabolism from causing cell damage. In children, it is important in preventing and treating skin conditions as well as boosting immunity.

Studies have reported that vitamin E protects against some of the toxicity of ionizing radiation. Vitamin E may help to decrease the toxicity of certain chemotherapy drugs such as adriamycin, which has a potential of major toxicity to the heart. Vitamin E may decrease some of the harmful effects of solar radiation on the skin. It works well in conjunction with beta carotene. Vitamin E appears to have a stabilizing effect on the vascular system, normalizing many blood vessel problems. It is useful in decreasing leg cramps, especially those occurring at night. Vitamin E is also helpful in treating burns secondary to radiation therapy.

Whether from a natural or a synthetic source, all forms supply the body with at least some vitamin E activity.

Recent studies indicate that high levels of stored iron in the body (ferritin) are associated with a greater risk of heart disease and diabetes. High-dose vitamin E supplements can interfere with iron absorption, and iron destroys vitamin E in the body. Therefore, if one is taking an iron supplement, it is best to take it about twelve hours apart from vitamin E.

Zinc: An antioxidant nutrient necessary for protein synthesis, wound healing, the development of the reproductive organs, and male hormone activity. Zinc governs the contractility of muscles and is important for blood stability and the prevention of anemia. It also maintains the body's alkaline balance and is part of many free radical–scavenging enzyme systems (antioxidants) such as superoxide dismutase (SOD). Zinc deficiency may result in delayed sexual maturity, prolonged healing of wounds, white spots on fingernails, retarded growth, stretch marks, fatigue, decreased alertness, and a greater susceptibility to infections.

Step Four: Control of Environmental Toxicity

Basic ways to control toxicity in your child's environment:

- Remove the source of any toxic materials such as stored or leaking chemicals, insecticides, cleaning agents, dyes, paints, solvents, glues, or acids.
- Use an effective air purification system.
- Replace furnace and air-conditioner filters regularly.
- Install a home water purification system (reverse osmosis or distilled); toxic chemicals can enter the body not only orally but through the skin and lungs when bathing or showering.
- Use baking soda to get rid of chemical odors—it neutralizes acid.
- Don't use scented fabric softeners.
- Avoid soft plastics; use ceramic, glass, or wood for bowls and storage; use cellophane bags instead of plastic whenever possible.
- Avoid room deodorants; improve ventilation instead.
- Avoid the use of insecticides, which can cause neurological impairment.

Removing Xenobiotics

Children accumulate the chemicals of our polluted world (xenobiotics) in their bodies' fat or muscle cells. These stored toxins can have many deleterious effects on health. The toxins can be slowly removed from the body by one or more of the following methods, depending on the severity of the problem:

- Bio-oxidative therapies such as ozone, hydrogen peroxide, and hyperbaric oxygen
- Chelation therapy
- Exercise
- Liver detoxification boosting (supplemental vitamins, minerals, and herbs)
- Normalizing circulatory, intestinal, and hormonal systems (depending on objective tests)
- Normalizing the nutritional state, especially fatty acid balances (depending on current status)
- Sauna

All these treatments are best administered in a controlled clinical setting, preferably by a doctor or clinic specializing in environmental medicine (formerly known as clinical ecology).

Dust Control

For those with severe allergies or sensitivities to dust, here are some basic measures to take:

- Remove all carpets and rugs; they hold dust and mold and may give off chemical fumes.
- Avoid heavy draperies that collect dust.
- Avoid wall pennants and other dust-catchers.
- Remove stuffed toys, stuffed furniture, pets, flowers, and plants from the room.
- Use simple wooden chairs and other items of furniture.
- Repair and seal heating ducts to keep dust out of the furnace.
- Heat rooms with electric heaters and cool using window air conditioners. This is very important for children with mold

allergies and children with severe allergies to environmental toxins. Healthy children probably do not need such measures.

- Clean the room frequently, using nontoxic, natural cleaning materials.
- Use a one-hundred-percent cotton mattress and avoid plastic covers to minimize chemical odors.
- Use one-hundred-percent cotton pillow filling, pillowcases, sheets, and pajamas.
- Change air-purification and air-conditioner filters frequently.
- Clean and vacuum the house while your child is away.
- Use an air purifier.

Mold Control

Molds are aggravating factors for many childhood illnesses. They thrive in cool, damp, and poorly ventilated areas, including refrigerators, garbage pails, basements, damp bathrooms, and under sinks. Here are some measures that help minimize the mold population in the home:

- Clean mold-prone areas frequently with Borax or Zephirain (available from pharmacies).
- Clean air conditioners, humidifiers, dehumidifiers, and vaporizers scrupulously.
- Clean behind wallpaper and paneling before installation, and under carpets and carpet pads.
- Get rid of synthetic carpets because they encourage mold growth; use cotton or wool rugs and clean them often.
- Clean mold-infested nooks and crannies in the bathroom, drains, laundry hamper, and towel hamper; regularly clean washcloths, damp towels, and all crevices.
- Keep the bathroom dry with an exhaust fan or open window.
- Keep the basement dry and seal cracks in the walls or floors.

- Use a dehumidifier.
- Keep ventilation and lighting optimal to discourage mold growth.
- Put crushed rock on top of house plant soil, as soil can provide a haven for molds; better still, keep plants outside or give them away.
- Frequently wash bedding and mattresses or throw them out if mold infestation cannot be eliminated.
- Throw away old magazines and newspapers.
- Bring more sunlight into your home (e.g., remove shrubs or prune plants close to the house). If you live in a shaded area or near rivers or streams, your mold risk may be very high.
- Limit your child's outdoor mold exposure, such as might occur when raking leaves, mowing grass, or playing in hay.
- If possible, use an air purifier and have your child wear an allergy mask.

Chemical Control

Chemicals are everywhere and difficult for most children to avoid or adapt to successfully in any way. Whether a child develops symptoms from these chemicals depends on a number of variables including inherited tendency, the total load of chemical exposure, the child's nutritional state, how well the immune system is functioning, and the load of other allergenic exposure such as foods, pollens, and molds. The chemicals that most commonly affect children and cause coughing, sneezing, irritated eyes, sore membranes, muscle aches, irritability, and hyperactivity are:

adhesive tape

bath oils

cedar-scented furniture polish

chemical food colorings and preservatives

cleaning agents

clothing dyes

cosmetics

detergents

diesel fumes

disinfectants

formaldehyde

garbage fumes

hair sprays

inks

insecticides: moth balls, insect repellents, Chlordane

knotty pine odors

marking pencils

nail polish

natural gas

paints, varnishes, shellac

petroleum products such as gasoline

pine-scented deodorants

plastics

polishes

synthetic textiles such as dacron, orlon, polyester, rayon

tobacco smoke

waxes

7

Natural Treatments for Other Allergy-Connected Illnesses

> Health is not simply the absence of disease but a state of complete
> well-being.
>
> —*World Health Organization*

As a group, our children are the sickest they have been in the history of the human species. Many scientists believe that this is because we continually poison our environment with the seventy thousand chemicals (four billion tons) in use at the present time. On top of that, we add two thousand new ones every year. Mercury, aluminum, lead, cadmium, and arsenic are just a few of the many toxins building up to dangerous levels in the bodies of our children, thanks to modern technology.

The dominant chronic problems of children in the late 1990s are epidemics of altered immunity, chronic fatigue, food and chemical allergies, chemical sensitivities, environmentally induced illnesses, chronic headaches, joint and muscle disorders, recurrent viral infections, blood sugar control problems, autoimmune diseases, and mood, behavior, and memory problems.

These medical problems are all preventable, controllable, and even curable with complementary medical therapeutics. With the exception of emergency care, conventional medicine, with its emphasis on symptom suppression and drug use, is virtually useless in dealing with contemporary childhood illnesses. This chapter presents information on more viable and effective therapies to help reverse common, chronic childhood illnesses.

Alternative Therapy for Autoimmune Diseases: General Principles

A healthy immune system recognizes a foreign organism as being foreign through the action of specific receptors which identify only certain molecules (antigens) on the foreign surface. Certain health circumstances (see Chapter 1) can cause a child's immune system to recognize itself as foreign. This is called autoimmunity, an immune system reaction to one's own tissues, and results in autoimmune disease.

Autoimmune diseases can be:

- genetically inherited
- caused by foreign chemicals (xenobiotics)
- caused by heavy metals (mercury, cadmium, lead, aluminum, arsenic, etc.)
- caused by digestive system abnormalities such as the leaky gut syndrome
- caused by abnormal tissues in the body such as a tumor, parasites, or fungi (candida)
- caused by emotional or psychological stressors from often unsuspected sources

Autoimmune diseases in children:

- AIDS (acquired immune deficiency syndrome)
- anemia (hemolytic, antoimmune type)
- arthritis (juvenile rheumatoid type)
- asthma
- dermatitis herpetiformis
- diabetes mellitus, insulin-dependent
- encephalomyelitis, allergic

- encephalomyelitis, myalgic (also known as chronic fatigue syndrome)
- generalized eczema
- glomerulonephritis (membranous type)
- nephrotic syndrome
- psoriasis
- vitiligo

Pro-inflammatory mediators in the body (e.g., histamine, some prostaglandins, and leukotrienes) are associated with autoimmune diseases. These mediators are thought by scientists to be responsible for pain, swelling, redness, and eventual scarring reactions such as fibrosis in the body. Prednisone, prednisolone, dexamethasone, and betamethasone are commonly prescribed anti-inflammatory corticosteroid drugs used to block the pro-inflammatory mediators and offset some of their more serious effects. Corticosteroid pills or creams are often prescribed for these conditions as well.

Although prednisone and other steroid drugs are effective at reducing inflammation, this comes at a huge price. These drugs cripple the immune system if taken for long periods of time. Some of the more common side effects include weight gain, fluid retention, increased appetite, increased risk of infection, depression, high blood pressure, diabetes, ulcers, acne, weak muscles, osteoporosis, insomnia, and an increased risk of blood clots.

The Natural Approach to Autoimmune Disease

It must be stressed that, in emergency, acute autoimmune disease flare-ups (asthmatic crisis, diabetic ketoacidosis, septicemia, etc.), drugs such as prednisone, intravenous antibiotics, and other anti-inflammatory drugs are lifesaving. Natural therapies do not have a place here.

All autoimmune diseases will wax and wane, periodically going closer to remission (fewer symptoms and less medication required for no obvious reason). It is at times like these that a natural, complementary approach can be taken to reduce the dependence on steroid and other drugs and to, in some cases, reverse the disease in question completely. Do not attempt any of this with your child without the supervision of a licensed health care practitioner. Such a person can prescribe and supervise the following steps in helping your child deal with auto-immune disease naturally:

Detection of food and chemical allergies: This is ideally done by a combination of elimination-provocation (exclusion diet) techniques and blood tests, such as the ELISA/Act test or other RAST blood tests. These blood tests are often misleading if the child is taking prednisone or aspirin. Usually, the child must be off prednisone for several weeks before blood tests for hidden food allergies can be determined. The elimination diet (see Chapter 2) is probably the best tool in such cases.

The use of natural fatty acid anti-inflammatory supplements: The type of fat found exclusively in meats and dairy products is known as arachidonic acid. Saturated animal fats and arachidonic acid increase the inflammatory response by stimulating the production of inflammatory prostaglandins and leukotrienes.

Vegetarian diets that avoid dairy products and eggs and use flaxseed, salmon oil, evening primrose oil, borage oil, olive oil, and black currant seed oil are higher in the essential fatty acids (EFAs)—linoleic and linolenic acids—which stimulate the synthesis of anti-inflammatory prostaglandins.

Another way to obtain anti-inflammatory essential fatty acids from the diet is to consume more cold-water fish such as salmon, trout, mackerel, sardines, swordfish, shark, cod, and halibut. These fish contain high concentrations of omega-3 fatty acids, which have also been documented to blunt the inflammatory or allergic response. If fish is either unpalatable for the individual or not readily available, supplementation with nine to twelve grams of EFAs daily from oil capsules is an alternative.

If diarrhea develops as a side effect of oil supplementation, reduce the dosage to tolerable levels. Also, vitamin E supplementation is important whenever a person takes essential fatty acid supplements because the polyunsaturated essential fatty acids quickly become peroxidized. In children, daily dosages of vitamin E as high as 3,000 IU have given good anti-inflammatory results.

Supplementation with antioxidants: Since the inflammatory response creates oxidative damage to tissues, the use of antioxidants helps prevent tissue damage that leads to permanent dysfunction. Antioxidant supplements include vitamins C, E, and B complex; coenzyme Q10; the natural carotenoids (carotenes, lycopenes, and others); bioflavonoids such as rutin, hesperidin, quercetin, catechin, and the proanthocyanidins (grape-seed extract, pine-bark extract, bilberry, and others); the minerals selenium and zinc; hormones such as DHEA (dehydoepiandosterone) and melatonin; and sulfur-containing amino acids such as cysteine, N-acetyl-cysteine, methionine, and glutathione. (See Chapter 6 for more information on antioxidants.)

Enzymes and other phytochemicals found in superfoods such as spirulina, chlorella, barley green, green kamut, bee pollen, royal jelly, and many herbs discussed later in this section are all potent antioxidants. Whole-leaf aloe vera juice with high MPS (mucopolysaccharide) content also contains high levels of dozens of natural antioxidants.

Some studies indicate that high doses of vitamin C and bioflavonoids are helpful in the treatment of many autoimmune conditions. Bioflavonoids such as rutin, hesperidin, catechin, quercetin, eriodictyol, pycnogenol, and grape-seed extract in high doses help strengthen the walls of capillaries, thereby preventing bruising (purpura). They stabilize the mast cell membranes and thus block the series of reactions that are associated with almost any allergy.

Bioflavonoids are found in many foods including citrus fruits (the white material just beneath the peel), onions, garlic, peppers, buckwheat, and black currants. In supplemental form, they have been successfully used for many years as a treatment for pain, bumps, bruises, and more severe athletic injuries. Bioflavonoids work together with vitamin C to protect blood vessels. They are also useful in the treatment of asthma and other allergic conditions which seemingly "only respond to antihistamines or steroids." Side effects of bioflavonoid supplementation in even megadoses are extremely rare.

Supplementation with natural anti-inflammatory enzymes and herbs: Pancreatin (animal-based pancreatic digestive enzymes), plant enzymes, and bromelain (from pineapples) not only help with protein digestion in the gastrointestinal tract but have been demonstrated to work as anti-inflammatory substances. They help reduce the number of pro-inflammatory chemical mediators like some prostaglandins and leukotrienes.

Curcumin is the yellow pigment of the herb turmeric. In some studies it has been reported to be as effective as cortisone without any of the associated side effects. Curcumin is primarily used as a natural anti-inflammatory agent, but it also has important applications in cancer prevention, antioxidant support, and the treatment of liver disorders, heart disease, and irritable bowel syndrome.

Trial therapies with antifungal regimes: Autoimmune diseases often respond to antifungal treatments. Evidence now exists that fungi, through their production of mycotoxins, initiate many autoimmune diseases by triggering inflammation in the gastrointestinal tract, which leads to the development of the leaky gut syndrome (see Chapter 1). The major killer diseases in North America are intimately connected to fungal mycotoxins.

Diseases of "unknown etiology" also often have a fungal connection, with treatment of the fungal infection bringing about an improvement or elimination of that disease.

In treating any fungal infection, it is important to realize that many foods which we have always considered to be health-providing have also been discovered to be heavily colonized by fungi and their mycotoxins. These include corn, peanuts, cashews, and dried coconuts. To a lesser degree, fungi can also be found in most breads and cereal grains. A diet high in contaminated grains and nuts increases the likelihood of fungal colonization of the gastrointestinal tract. Worse, animals fed mycotoxin-contaminated grains end up with fungal overgrowth. This is evidenced by the fact that the fat and muscles of most grain-fed animals in North America are loaded with mycotoxins. The association between animal fat and both heart disease and cancer is well documented; some researchers say that it's the mycotoxin load found in the animal fat that increases the risk.

The manufacture of bread, beer, wine, cheese, chewing tobacco, aged and cured meats, and cigarettes involves a fungal fermentation process which increases the likelihood of exposure to mycotoxins. The consumption of small amounts of these foods may be tolerated by those with healthy immune systems but can be deadly to those suffering from chronic illness of any kind.

Diet is very important in the treatment of any fungal infection. Sugar feeds fungi and must be eliminated from the diet. This includes maple syrup, honey, molasses, and fruit juice. In severe infections, even whole fruits should be eliminated for several weeks. Milk, white flour products, peanuts, mushrooms, melons, moldy foods (leftovers), and foods containing yeast all contribute to worsening any fungal infection. The ideal diet for fighting fungi can be found in books such as the *Complete Candida Yeast Guidebook* by Jeanne Marie Martin and this author (see Further Reading section).

Tea tree oil is derived from the Australian tree *Melaleucea alternifolia*. It has a variety of antimicrobial activities and has been used successfully in the treatment of many skin conditions, especially those associated with fungi or candida. Despite what you might read on the bottle label, tea tree oil is effective as a systemic antifungal remedy when swallowed with some water. The usual effective dose is about fifteen drops in water swallowed three times daily. Other effective antifungal oils taken internally are flaxseed oil, oregano oil, olive oil, borage oil, castor bean oil, evening primrose oil, and fish oils.

Other natural antifungal remedies are garlic, caprylic acid, echinacea, colloidal silver, and whole-leaf aloe vera juice. Taken internally, these can kill most harmful bacteria and fungi without significant side effects. Rare individuals respond poorly to the natural approach and are only helped by prescription antifungal drugs.

If there are enough "friendly" bacteria in the body, fungi are less likely to grow. Taking a regular supplement of *lactobacillus acidophilus* helps normalize the immune system.

Hormonal and other therapies: Autoimmune diseases have also been reported to respond to the hormone DHEA (dehydroepiandrosterone). DHEA is the most abundant androgen (male hormone) produced by the adrenal cortex of both males and females. It can be found in almost any organ, including the testes, the ovaries, the lungs, and the brain. Testosterone is synthesized from DHEA in both males and females. One theory as to why males get autoimmune diseases significantly less often than females is because of their relatively higher levels of DHEA and testosterone. Nutritional doctors have used DHEA in the treatment of fatigue, obesity, loss of libido, allergies, autoimmune diseases, stress, and hypoglycemia with varying degrees of success. In Canada and the United States, DHEA is available only on a doctor's prescription. Natural precursors to DHEA can be found in wild yam, but studies do not indicate that this is equivalent to the pure hormone.

Vitamin E may have little or no effect on autoimmune disease in low doses (under 1,200 IU per day). But in doses well above 2,000 IU, vitamin E weakens autoimmune disease and provides anti-inflammatory effects. Herbs such as aloe vera, burdock, comfrey, licorice root, white willow bark, curcumin (from turmeric), feverfew, devil's claw, yarrow, yucca, and marshmallow may also be helpful. Doses of all these supplemental nutrients have to be carefully individualized. Supervision by a nutritional medical doctor or a naturopath is highly advisable.

More Allergy-Connected Childhood Illnesses

Some of the following childhood illnesses, such as asthma and rhinitis, are known by most parents to be allergy-related. What is generally not known about these disorders is that they can often be reversed naturally, while boosting the child's resistance to disease.

Other illnesses covered in this section, such as epilepsy and depression, are not generally associated with autoimmunity or food or chemical allergies. My experience with all of them, however, leads me to conclude that this belief is very often incorrect. I urge every parent with a chronically ill child, especially one who has not responded well to conventional drug treatment, to look into these safe and effective alternatives.

Allergic Rhinitis

Allergic rhinitis (hay fever) occurs in six million children and accounts for two million days lost from school. It can be perennial or may occur only in the spring or fall, with symptoms such as sneezing, a clear nasal discharge, nasal stuffiness, and nasal itching. There may also be headaches, itching of the throat or soft palate, and postnasal drainage causing frequent throat clearing and a dry cough or hoarseness. Children suffering from allergic rhinitis appear to have a constant cold. The child may also develop habitual mouth-breathing and black discoloration under the eyes, called "allergic shiners."

One complication of perennial allergic rhinitis is otitis media, with an accumulation of fluid behind the eardrum (effusion). There may be loss of hearing, a sensation of fullness in the head, or popping and cracking noises.

Allergic rhinitis is conventionally treated with antihistamines, decongestants, steroid nasal sprays, anti-inflammatory drugs, allergy desensitization injections, or corticosteroid inhalers. Such treatments may sometimes do more harm than good. For example, the May 1993 issue of the *Townsend Letter for Doctors* reports that in the year 1991, there were 2,669 poisonings associated with the use of prescription analgesics, 412 with antihistamines, 953 with antimicrobials, 257 with asthma therapies, 1,526 with cough and cold preparations, and 619 with gastrointestinal drugs. In the same year, on the other hand, there were no poisonings reported with any vitamin, mineral, herb, or homeopathic remedy.

For each drug used to treat allergies, there is a corresponding natural remedy that often works better and with fewer side effects. Studies from around the world indicate that green foods (e.g., spirulina, chlorella, and blue-green algae) and bee pollen are effective treatments for allergies and help prevent recurrent infections and other allergy-associated conditions. Some scientists have called these supplements nature's most perfect foods.

One can achieve a very impressive antihistaminic effect in children by using high doses of vitamin C and bioflavonoids. Vitamin C should be started at low doses and gradually increased to the point where the child develops some diarrhea. The dose should then be lowered to match bowel tolerance. At this dosage level, vitamin C works as well as any prescription or over-the-counter antihistamine. Most children get good antihistaminic effects somewhere between 6,000 and 12,000 mg daily. As the symptoms clear, the vitamin C dosages can be reduced gradually.

Bioflavonoids, especially from the proanthocyanidin family (pycnogenols) prevent the release of the pro-inflammatory chemicals from the mast cell. They stabilize the mast cell membrane. As a result, rhinitis and the cold symptoms disappear. The optimal dose is the lowest one which prevents the rhinitis. For some children, this is 300 mg daily. For others, it might be just 25 mg. The use of both bioflavonoids and vitamin C to bowel tolerance is best prescribed and supervised by a qualified natural health practitioner.

Studies have also shown that refined carbohydrates (glucose, fructose, and sucrose) have a depressant effect on the immune system as early as an hour after eating them. Removing sugar and white flour products from the diet is often helpful with most of the signs and symptoms of allergies. A diet high in saturated animal fats impairs immune function. A higher intake of the omega-3 EPA oils (found in halibut, cod, mackerel, salmon, trout, tuna, and many other fish) and gamma linolenic acid (flaxseed oil or edible linseed oil, evening primrose oil, oil of borage, black currant oil, etc.) enhances immune function. More often than not, essential fatty acid supplementation alone reverses the symptoms of many chronic allergy conditions.

Other natural supplements that have been documented to lessen allergies in children include the very potent bioflavonoid pycnogenol and common herbs such as echinacea, goldenseal, elderberry, capsicum, horehound, chamomile, calendula, taheebo (*pau d'arco*), garlic, astragalus, hypericum, and lomatium. Some children with severe allergies may benefit from anticandida treatments such as *lactobacillus acidophilus*, garlic, tea tree oil, olive oil, caprylic acid, castor bean oil, evening primrose oil, digestive enzymes, and others.

Childhood Junk Food Addictions

Children and sugar are sometimes difficult to separate. Some children are so addicted to sweets that they will hunt all over the house until their cravings are satisfied. Some will display aggressive or antisocial behavior to get chocolates or candy bars. Addictions of all kinds, including those to sugar and junk food, can be overcome with the help of nutritional therapies. Although most mainstream health professionals believe that only psychotherapy, behavior modification, or prescription drugs can eliminate addictions, a growing number of people are seeing the importance of rebalancing biochemistry in children with these chronic problems.

It is well known that addicts suffer from a long list of nutritional deficiencies because of the depleting effects of the addictive substance on nutrient reserves. Hidden food or chemical allergies are behind many cases of addiction, and improvement is often seen within a few weeks after elimination of offending substances from the diet or the environment. One should see a natural health care practitioner for a comprehensive nutritional and biochemical assessment before starting on drastic diet changes and food supplements.

If I had to recommend only a few supplements for treating addictions which could really do no harm, I would first suggest using a broad-spectrum antioxidant combination product. Second, a broad-spectrum, hypoallergenic amino acid supplement, a good B complex vitamin, and a multimineral supplement (perferably colloidal minerals in a liquid form) will help cut cravings for low-nutrient junk food. Bee pollen powder, aloe vera juice, and beet root powder are additional options that provide strong nutrient support against addictions.

Natural hormones such as melatonin might also be effective therapy since many children indulge their addictions in order to elevate melatonin, and hence serotonin, levels in the brain. Excessive consumption of alcohol, caffeine, aspirin, sugar, or drugs depletes melatonin reserves in the body.

Canker Sores

Canker sores (aphthous ulcers) are tiny ulcerations that occur in the oral cavity, on or near the tongue. They can be quite painful, to the point of interfering with eating. The source of the problem is usually an acid condition in the body caused by food allergies or a virus. Some children are more prone to canker sores, especially if they have a history of heavy antibiotic use or diets high in sugar and white flour products. Suboptimal immune systems are almost always involved.

The first thing one should do is eliminate strongly acid foods such as citrus fruits, tomatoes, red meats, and processed foods. It's best to avoid all fruits, with the possible exception of bananas. Supplementation of the diet with calcium carbonate or calcium aspartate will also help buffer the acid condition, as will *lactobacillus acidophilus* powder or capsules. If your child is taking vitamin C as a regular supplement, switch over to a buffered form such as sodium or calcium ascorbate or ester C.

An immediate remedy for canker sores is to take one-half teaspoon of sodium bicarbonate powder mixed with water four or more times a day. This can be used as a mouth rinse and can also be swallowed to help make the body more alkaline. Also, vitamin E capsules may be punctured and the liquid contents applied directly to the canker sores several times daily to speed healing.

A variety of commercial toothpastes containing sodium bicarbonate can be used instead of standard toothpastes high in fluoride and other chemicals which could iritate canker sores and increase pain.

Many children have also reported excellent relief of aphthous ulcers from tea tree oil mouth rinses and aqueous colloidal silver. Both have natural antimicrobial effects and boost immunity. Using either or both after brushing the teeth helps prevent any type of oral infection, including parasites and candida.

For a period of about two weeks, sufferers should also supplement with beta carotene, zinc picolinate, gamma linoleic acid (from evening primrose oil), L-lysine, and vitamin E. Zinc, by the way, is therapeutic for ulcers anywhere in the body; long-term use (over two weeks) should be balanced with copper supplementation.

Some children with canker sores also benefit from iron, vitamin B-12, and folic acid supplementation, in either oral or injected forms. Herbal remedies such as echinacea, goldenseal, taheebo, burdock, red clover, red raspberry, hypericum, aloe vera juice, and calendula are also frequently effective.

Poor dental hygiene, stress, and bowel abnormalities such as Crohn's disease may also lead to chronic canker sores. Candidiasis is secondary to these and other immune system abnormalities and may need to be treated in some stubborn cases. Symptoms of candida infection in the mouth include pain and a burning sensation. Abdominal gas, indigestion, and pain may also be signs of a yeast overgrowth in the large bowel. For more detailed information on candida problems, please refer to the *Complete Candida Yeast Guidebook* by Jeanne Marie Martin and this author.

Eczema

Eczema is a mildly painful and sometimes itchy inflammatory skin eruption which can occur on any part of the body. It is a common childhood problem which can be caused by stress and emotional factors, nutritional deficiencies, food allergies, and digestive abnormalities, including low stomach acid and low pancreatic enzyme levels. Dermatologists usually prescribe cortisone-based creams to treat eczema; they rarely consider the systemic source of a rash, preferring to suppress the symptoms.

For those who wish to adopt a more natural approach, diet should be as fresh and unrefined as possible. Avoid chemicals, animal products, processed foods, coffee, tea, alcohol, and sugar in any form. Even the sugar found naturally in fruit and fruit juices might aggravate chronic eczema in some children. Dairy products and eggs are strongly allergenic, and a several-week trial therapy of strict avoidance of these foods will do no harm. Animal products may also be loaded with drugs such as antibiotics, synthetic hormones, nitrates, nitrites, and other skin toxins. For short-term relief, an organic, plant-based diet is best. As symptoms improve, poultry and fish can be added back to the diet. Later, whole fresh fruits can be consumed on a trial basis. If the eczema returns upon reintroduction of any food, a stricter dietary approach of either complete avoidance or a four-day rotation of reaction-producing foods can be instituted.

Topically, calendula cream, vitamin E cream, and aloe vera gel aid healing and prevent infections.

Nutrient supplements that may be very helpful for both treatment and prevention include essential fatty acids (e.g., salmon oil, evening primrose oil, flaxseed oil, black currant seed oil, oil of borage, etc.), vitamin A, B complex vitamins including biotin, vitamin C, bioflavonoids (pycnogenol, hesperidin, catechin, quercetin), vitamin E, zinc, calendula, tea tree oil, and aloe vera. Treatment depends mainly on biochemical individuality, which can be determined by professional consultation and testing. See a naturopath or a medical doctor familiar with the natural approach for a program personalized to your child.

Childhood Chronic Fatigue

Chronic fatigue or tiredness is a symptom that often brings children of all ages to a doctor. Only twenty percent of these children have a diagnosable or treatable medical condition, while the remainder have no obvious physical source of their chronic weariness or exhaustion. My experience is that virtually all of these children have delayed food allergies to commonly eaten foods such as wheat, milk, yeast, and eggs.

An indeterminate percentage of these cases is related to a virus, as in chronic fatigue syndrome (also called myalgic encephalomyelitis, or ME; see further discussion following). In the majority of cases, however, no specific cause is established, and treatment is largely through trial and error using a variety of drugs. What can one do when conventional doctors have ruled out cancer, diabetes, heart disease, hypothyroidism, and other metabolic disorders as possible causes of chronic fatigue? Are there any alternatives to just accepting it as a phase or a psychosomatic disturbance?

Self-Help Measures

Although the following measures are best taken with the guidance of a natural health care practitioner, their safety is high enough for most parents to attempt them with their child without supervision:

Revise the diet: There is an inverse relationship between chronic fatigue and the health of the immune system. Since sugar suppresses immunity, eliminate it in all its forms, including the milk sugar lactose. Avoid cheese, grain-fed animal products (red meats, especially beef and pork, animal fats, milk, and other high-fat dairy products), refined foods, and caffeine-containing products, including soft drinks. Avoid feeding your child leftovers or allowing him or her to be exposed to tobacco smoke.

Eliminate shortening, lard, margarine, beef tallow, and fried foods in general. Instead, use more fish and fish oils, garlic, onions, olives, olive oil, green vegetables, herbs, spices, soy products, yogurt, psyllium, pectin, and milled (ground) flaxseed, provided that these foods don't produce symptoms. An increased intake of fiber significantly reduces the impact of toxins found in many commercial foods.

Supplement the diet with energy-boosting herbs and other concentrated nutrients:

- Whole-food concentrates such as bee pollen, beet root powder, royal jelly, kelp, dulse, spirulina, chlorella, barley green, and aloe vera juice have a naturally high vitamin and mineral content with highly bioavailable antioxidants. They are also low in calories, fats, salts, and sugar and high in live active enzymes and soluble fiber. They are a convenient way of supplying the vital five daily servings of fruits and vegetables.

• Herbal teas, capsules, or tinctures that boost energy and enhance a general sense of well-being include *ma huang* (ephedra), *ginkgo biloba,* Siberian ginseng, ginger, *yerba maté,* kola nut, *fo-ti,* and licorice root.

• Vitamin and mineral supplements that are helpful in combating fatigue include B complex vitamins (especially vitamins B-1, B-5, B-6, and B-12), vitamin C, zinc, copper, manganese, chromium, and magnesium.

• Other nutrient supplements have energy-enhancing properties, especially coenzyme Q10, pycnogenols, *lactobacillus acidophilus* and *bifido* bacteria, and amino acids such as carnitine, taurine, tyrosine, and phenylalanine.

How a Health Care Practitioner Can Help

The following diagnostic and treatment possibilities are often worth investigating, especially for children whose chronic fatigue fails to respond to medical intervention or the simple self-help measures discussed earlier. Discuss these possibly overlooked diagnoses and treatment options with your natural health care practitioner.

• Low-grade depression, often accompanied by anxiety. It should not be forgotten that insomnia, fatigue, eating disorders, memory loss, and multiple intractable somatic complaints are common symptoms of a clinical depression even in children. This diagnosis is usually the most resisted by chronically fatigued victims, but psychotherapy may well be worth a try. Other treatment options include aerobic exercise, breathing exercises, massage therapy, acupressure, or shiatsu, and other relaxation techniques suitable for children.

• Subclinical hypothyroidism, or Wilson's disease (body temperatures are consistently below 98.6°F or 37°C). In such cases, fatigue usually responds to supplementation with natural thyroid hormone precursors such as iodine, tyrosine, zinc, copper, and selenium or to thyroid hormone itself (i.e., desiccated thyroid or liothyronine). In children, subclinical hypothyroidism can almost always be reversed simply by eliminating sugar and refined carbohydrates.

- Toxic heavy-metal excess or hypersensitivity—especially a sensitivity to mercury in dental amalgams, but also to lead, cadmium, aluminum, copper, arsenic, and nickel. Ridding the body of these toxins through a variety of natural supplements such as garlic, N-acetyl-cysteine, vitamin C, vitamin E, and selenium often eliminates fatigue. Such supplementation should be supervised. In more severe cases, intravenous chelation therapy is effective.

- Vitamin deficiencies, especially of B complex vitamins. In particular, folic acid and vitamin B-12 may be poorly absorbed in the intestines of chronically ill individuals. Injections of vitamin B-12 and folic acid may be necessary until gut healing can take place.

- Mineral deficiencies or imbalances involving iron, zinc, copper, selenium, calcium, magnesium, chromium, manganese, silicon, boron, iodine, and lithium. Iron deficiency is not the only mineral deficiency capable of causing fatigue; testing for other mineral deficiencies may be important.

- Essential fatty acid and amino acid deficiencies due to malabsorption caused by digestive enzyme deficiencies. Amino acids are precursors to all the neurotransmitters responsible for optimal brain and nervous system function. Essential fatty acids are important components of all body cells and particularly vital for the health of the nervous system.

- Masked or delayed food allergies or chemical hypersensitivities that can only be determined by elimination-provocation testing or blood tests such as RAST or ELISA.

- Hypoglycemia or hyperglycemia due to endocrine gland dysfunction other than the thyroid (pancreas, adrenal, gonadal disease). Blood levels of hormones such as DHEA, cortisol, and insulin might all be at suboptimal levels.

• Chronic candida, fungal infection, or hypersensitivity syndrome. This is best diagnosed and treated by a trial therapy with a sugar-free, yeast-free diet and natural antifungal supplements such as garlic, taheebo, tea tree oil, colloidal silver, olive oil, *acidophilus,* and others.

• Chronic parasitic infestations. These are associated not only with digestive problems such as chronic constipation or diarrhea, but with chronic fatigue and immune system malfunctions of nearly every type.

• Low stomach acidity or low pancreatic enzyme production. This can lead to subclinical malabsorption syndromes and numerous nutrient deficiencies which, when corrected, alleviate some cases of chronic fatigue.

Chronic Fatigue Syndrome

Neurasthenia and myalgic encephalomyelitis (ME) are two names for the debilitating flu-like illness best known as chronic fatigue syndrome (CFS). It was first described in medical literature in 1869, corresponding to the beginning of the industrial revolution. At one time, the cause was thought to be the Epstein-Barr virus, but this has been disproven and the exact etiology is still unknown. About fifteen percent of the general population and an undetermined number of children now suffer from CFS.

CFS is a complex illness characterized by incapacitating fatigue (exhaustion and extremely poor stamina), neurological problems, and a constellation of symptoms resembling other disorders such as mononucleosis, multiple sclerosis, fibromyalgia, AIDS-related complex (ARC), Lyme disease, post-polio syndrome, and autoimmune diseases such as lupus. The symptoms tend to wax and wane but are often severely debilitating and may last for many months or years.

CFS victims tend to be far more sensitive to prescription medications than the average person, with a high probability of having side effects to antidepressants, antibiotics, and even herbal, vitamin, and mineral remedies. Common to most victims is a frustration with the conventional medical system and insurance companies, which refuse to accept the validity of the diagnosis.

In 1985, the CDC (Centers for Disease Control) formulated a set of criteria for the diagnosis of what it called chronic fatigue syndrome, which is now called chronic fatigue and immunodysfunction syndrome (CFIDS). To meet the CDC definition, a child must fulfill two "major criteria" and either eight of eleven "symptom criteria" or six of the symptom criteria and two of three "physical criteria."

The major criteria are:

1. New onset of persistent or relapsing, debilitating fatigue or easy loss of energy, in a child who has no previous history of similar symptoms, that does not resolve with bed rest and that is severe enough to reduce or impair average daily activity below fifty percent of the child's premorbid activity level for a period of at least six months.
2. New onset of cognitive dysfunction with short-term memory loss, confusion, disorientation, sequencing dysfunction, word searching or recall problems, diminished comprehension of oral or written information, problems with calculations, and difficulties in processing, maintaining, or expressing thoughts.
3. Exclusion of other plausible disorders by thorough evaluation based on history, physical examination, and appropriate laboratory findings.

The CDC's symptom criteria include onset of the symptom complex over a few hours or days and ten other symptoms which must be documented on at least two occasions, at least one month apart:

1. Fever and/or chills.
2. Sore, scratchy, relapsing throat problem.
3. Lymphatic soreness or swelling in at least two sites.

4. Muscle discomfort, flu-like muscle aches, muscles sore to the touch.
5. Fibromyalgia with eight out of eighteen classic tender spots.
6. Generalized weakness.
7. Joint discomfort: migratory and asymmetrical, involving large joints more than small ones.
8. Headache: new-onset pressure type, behind the eyes (retro-orbital) and occipital, that worsens with stress and exertion.
9. Sleep disturbances and hypersomnolence (ten hours of sleep per night plus naps).
10. Chronic frequent nausea.

Despite research that proves otherwise, many patients I have seen in the past year are still being told by doctors that CFS is a form of depression or that "it's all in your head." CFS is not just a psychiatric illness. Antidepressant drugs are usually ineffective. There are many illnesses that have chronic fatigue as a major symptom, including depression, autoimmune disease, environmental illness, and other types of viral illness. All of these illnesses share a similar type of molecular damage from oxidative stress.

Chronic fatigue syndrome cannot be understood through the simplistic single-agent, single-disease medical model. One must look at a more holistic picture that includes biochemistry and the environmental influences of invading organisms, allergies, chemical and heavy-metal damage, digestive abnormalities, nutritional (antioxidant, etc.) deficiencies, and the stresses of modern life. Unfortunately, there is no simple lab test to determine a diagnosis of CFS. A psychological test called the MMPI (Minnesota Multiphasic Personality Inventory) shows a specific pattern of test scores to be associated with organic disease identical to CFS and not found in any other disorder. This test, however, is not universally considered diagnostic for CFS.

CFS results from a dysfunction of the immune system which can generally be understood as a disease of autoimmunity. In many children with CFS there are functional deficiencies in natural killer cells—an important component of the immune system responsible for protection against viruses. Many scientists believe that viruses may be directly involved in causing the initial injury to the immune system. These viruses include entero-viruses, herpes viruses (especially human herpes virus-6, or HHV-6), and retroviruses. Whether or not a child develops CFS is believed to be a function of how his or her system deals with the causative agent(s). CFS is not considered contagious, since most people in close contact with CFS patients do not develop the illness.

Treatment

There is no specific conventional medical treatment for CFS other than rest, analgesics, and other symptomatic measures. It is important and even therapeutic to keep an open mind about CFS and not listen to negative people, medical or otherwise, who claim that nothing can be done or that the child should see a psychiatrist. All cases of CFS improve or completely resolve with time (from a few months to a few years). This is not the case in adults, many of who suffer from debilitating fatigue for a decade or longer after the diagnosis is made. Recovery rates are highly variable and very difficult to predict but can be enhanced by complementary medical approaches.

The immune system requires healthy levels of all the essen-tial amino acids, zinc, calcium, magnesium, potassium, sele-nium, germanium, silicon, iron, beta carotene, vitamin C, vitamin E, vitamin A, and B complex vitamins, especially vita-mins B-5, B-6, and B-12, just to name a few. Amino acid analysis, hair mineral analysis, and live-cell microscopy are just a few of the many tests on nutritional status which can often help chil-dren open the doors to a speedier recovery.

Studies have also shown that refined carbohydrates (glu-cose, fructose, and sucrose) have a depressant effect on the im-mune system as early as an hour after eating them. Removing sugar and white flour products from the diet is often helpful with most of the signs and symptoms of CFS.

A hypoallergenic rotation diet with seventy percent of the calories coming from complex carbohydrates (whole grains, fruits, vegetables, and legumes) is best. Avoidance of caffeine, alcohol, and processed foods is also important. If possible, get food allergy, candida, and chemical allergy testing done by the ELISA/Act blood test.

If your child has CFS and irritable bowel symptoms (constipation, bloating, gas, diarrhea, mucus discharge, etc.), ask your doctor to order a battery of tests called the CDSA (comprehensive digestive and stool analysis) combined with a CP (comprehensive parasitology). CFS victims often need help with digestive enzyme function, bowel flora balance, or infestations with parasites, candida, or other pathogenic microbes.

A higher dietary intake of the omega-3 EPA oils (found in halibut, cod, mackerel, salmon, trout, shark, and many other fish) and gamma linolenic acid (GLA) are of proven benefit to CFS sufferers. Despite what some say about the relative merits or drawbacks of the various GLA supplements (flaxseed or edible linseed oil, evening primrose oil, borage oil, black currant oil, etc.), I have noticed no significant difference in the immune-normalizing results obtained from one source as opposed to another. I recommend experimentation with the different GLA sources before deciding on any specific brand.

Several herbs and whole-food supplements are helpful to both boost immunity and control the symptoms of CFS. Some work better for given individuals than for others, so it's best to avoid generalizations and dogma about any natural treatments. Many doctors and CFS sufferers have reported good results with a long list of safe natural supplements, as found below.

Natural immune system boosters and CFS fighters:

adrenal extract

astragalus

baptisia

blue-green algae, barley green, spirulina, green kamut, and other whole green foods

burdock, slippery elm, sheep sorrel, and Turkish rhubarb combination

calendula

carnitine

cat's claw

chaparral

coenzyme Q10

colloidal silver

DHEA

DMG (dimethyl glycine)

echinacea

garlic

ginkgo biloba

goldenseal

hypericum (St. John's wort)

kelp, dulse, and other seaweeds

kola nut

lactobacillus acidophilus and *bifidus*

licorice

liothyronine

lomatium

ma huang

methionine

pau d'arco (taheebo)

phenylalanine

pokeweed

propolis, bee pollen, royal jelly

pycnogenol

red clover

shiitake mushroom

Siberian ginseng

thymus gland extract

tyrosine

whole-leaf aloe vera juice

yarrow

yerba maté

Homeopathic remedies such as Ignatia, Natrum muriaticum, cell salts, and Nux vomica often help CFS victims who are unable to tolerate vitamins, minerals, and herbs. Consultation with a homeopathic physician is highly recommended.

Epilepsy and Seizure Disorders

There are a number of natural therapies that can be considered as complementary medicine for the treatment of seizure disorders. The cause of seizures is often unknown. In some cases, they can be linked to infection, meningitis, head injuries, drugs, lack of oxygen, spasm in the blood vessels, immunizations, food allergies, or hereditary factors.

Nutrition does play a role, since seizures may also be associated with malnutrition, hidden food allergies, and hypoglycemia (low blood sugar). Recent research has linked both tremors and seizures with consumption of the natural sweetener aspartame. If aspartame is in the diet, replace it with a natural sweetener such as *stevia*, honey, or sucanat (see Chapter 1 for more information). Aluminum, mercury, and lead toxicity may also contribute to the problem; hair mineral analysis can determine whether levels of these toxic heavy metals are elevated in the body. Other biochemical tests, including live blood cell analysis, should be done to determine nutritional deficiencies. Food allergy testing can be done in a variety of ways, but the ELISA/Act test is preferred, since it does not rely on eliciting symptoms through food elimination and provocation, which could reproduce a seizure.

There are many reports of the benefits of certain nutritional supplements in the control of seizure disorders. These include the amino acids L-taurine, L-glutamine, L-tryptophan, and L-tyrosine. Also important are magnesium (this sometimes only works if injected intramuscularly), vitamin B-6, vitamin B-12, other B complex vitamins, calcium, zinc, chromium, manganese, selenium, essential fatty acids (evening primrose oil, flaxseed oil, oil of borage) and vitamins A, C, and E. Herbs such as valerian, hypericum, skullcap, lobelia, passion flower, gotu kola, and juniper berries might also be helpful. Melatonin—the popular natural remedy for sleep disorders—has recently been reported to help reverse epilepsy in some children. Melatonin might be working as a free radical scavenger, much like vitamin E, selenium, and glutathione.

The ketogenic diet, although generally not recommended for healthy children because of the highly acid state it produces, has been shown to help control seizure disorders in some children. The ketogenic diet (high fat, low protein, low carbohydrate) was popular as a treatment for seizures in the 1920s before anticonvulsant medications were available. For children starting out on this diet, the recommended ratio of fats to protein and carbohydrates combined is 4:1; it can usually be lowered to 3:1 after the first year. According to Dr. John M. Freeman, director of the Pediatric Epilepsy Clinic at Children's Center in Baltimore, Maryland, the high-fat ketogenic diet works "better than any other regimen" to control seizures in epileptic children. He recommends this diet for children who do not respond to anticonvulsant drugs. Some experts claim that this diet can reduce seizures by up to seventy percent, but approximately a third of those who start this diet do not tolerate its side effects of diarrhea and dehydration. Obviously, this diet is best followed under the supervision of a qualified health care practitioner.

Sample Ketogenic Diet

Day 1

Breakfast: Scrambled eggs, butter, diluted cream (to drink), orange juice.

Lunch: Lettuce leaf with mayonnaise, spaghetti squash with butter and Parmesan cheese, orange soda mixed with whipped cream.

Dinner: Asparagus with butter, chopped lettuce with mayonnaise, hot dog slices with ketchup, vanilla ice cream.

Day 2

Breakfast: Bacon, melon slices, scrambled eggs with butter, vanilla cream shake.

Lunch: Celery and cucumber sticks, tuna with mayonnaise, and jello with whipped cream.

Dinner: Chopped lettuce with mayonnaise, broiled chicken breasts, a cinnamon apple slice with butter topped with vanilla ice cream.

For more information, see Dr. John M. Freeman's book entitled *The Epilepsy Diet Treatment: An Introduction to the Ketogenic Diet.*

The ketogenic diet should only be attempted as a trial after food allergy testing has been done and the reactive (allergenic) foods have been eliminated, with no improvement. If seizures stop after the reactive foods have been eliminated, there is no reason to attempt the ketogenic diet. Because of the large number of children who will receive significant side effects on the ketogenic diet, it is best to leave this approach to childhood epilepsy as a last approach.

In general, this diet is contrary to the advice of most nutritional experts but seems to be effective with certain children who suffer from seizure disorders.

Complementary medical therapies that use a combination of diet changes and supplemental vitamins, minerals, and herbs are not always going to reverse a seizure disorder. They will, however, almost always improve the general health of the child and reduce his or her dependence on prescription drugs.

Muscle Spasms

Spasm of any kind—whether in the neck muscles causing headaches or in the muscles lining the bowel wall causing irritable bowel syndrome, proctalgia (rectal pain), or chronic diarrhea—is commonly caused by magnesium deficiency, hidden food and chemical allergies, or both. Calcium channel blockers are prescription drugs commonly used to treat angina, migraines, and other types of pain or spasm. They block the rapid influx of calcium into cells responsible for the symptoms. Since magnesium supplementation can do virtually the same thing, as well as reduce pain, spasm, or tremor, it has been dubbed nature's calcium channel blocker.

The usual causes of magnesium deficiency are stress, poor diet, and excessive use of caffeine (from chocolate or soft drinks). Depending on the severity of the deficiency, a lack of magnesium may result in muscle spasms, palpitations, high blood pressure, insomnia, irritability, anxiety, constipation, cramps, pain, and even seizures. There are various tests which can indicate whether a child's magnesium status is optimal. Red or white blood cell magnesium levels will probably indicate a deficiency, but they are not one hundred percent reliable. Hair mineral analysis may be more helpful, but it is not universally accepted as a legitimate way to assess magnesium status. The best test in many cases, aside from a magnesium loading test, is a trial therapy with magnesium supplementation or intramuscular magnesium injections.

One can improve magnesium levels by eating large amounts of raw greens and avoiding sugar, coffee, tea, cola drinks, chocolate, and pills that contain caffeine. There is no harm in doing this. If symptoms suddenly worsen as a result of this dietary change, it is very likely that the child has a masked allergy to what was eliminated from the diet. Adding these things back to the diet usually clears the symptoms but gives both parents and children the mistaken idea that they "need" caffeine, sugar, or chocolate. In reality, the worsening of symptoms triggered by the elimination of certain foods from the diet is a withdrawal reaction similar to those experienced by alcoholics or cigarette addicts when they give up alcohol or cigarettes. Withdrawal reactions to foods can sometimes be severe. They usually settle within four to seven days and can be eased by using a combination of bicarbonate powder and vitamin C.

Magnesium levels in the body can be enhanced by supplementing the diet with liquid chlorophyll and other green food supplements such as spirulina, chlorella, barley green, green magma, blue-green algae, and liquid or encapsulated magnesium citrate, aspartate, or gluconate. If your child has no kidney problems, taking even one hundred tablespoons of magnesium a day is safe. The body just gets rid of the excess through the kidneys and bowel. Watch for diarrhea as a possible side effect; if it occurs, reduce the dose of magnesium by half or more.

If you give your child magnesium in high doses, it's a good idea to include a vitamin B complex supplement daily that contains at least 100 mg of vitamin B-6. Magnesium and vitamin B-6 work synergistically for pain and spasm control. Follow this combined therapy for at least six weeks before deciding whether it is working.

If oral supplementation fails, magnesium sulfate injections will often stop spasms. The injections are given intramuscularly or intravenously at least twice weekly for six or more weeks. The dosage depends on the child's age and ranges from 500 mg to 1,500 mg per injection. Although these injections are usually given by doctors or naturopaths, nonmedical people can learn how to self-inject magnesium (or a parent can learn how to inject a child) and any other nutrient much the same way that diabetics can self-inject insulin on a daily basis.

In addition to magnesium and vitamin B-6, there are many natural supplements that can help alleviate irritability and spasm. These include calcium if calcium is deficient, potassium, zinc, brewer's yeast, lecithin, octacosanol, and vitamin E. It has recently been reported that melatonin, the naturally occurring pineal gland hormone, is effective in reducing spasms and seizures.

In people with low or absent stomach acid secretion, injections of B vitamins, especially vitamin B-12, can dramatically improve nervous system function, which can be related to spasm in any area. The same can be said for folic acid, a nutrient which, when deficient, can cause pain and nervous abnormalities such as the restless leg syndrome.

Herbal remedies such as chamomile, hops, lady slipper, passion flower, skullcap, wood betony, hypericum, and valerian in tea, capsule, or tincture form may also be of help in some cases. The herbal tonic called Salusan (from Flora Distributors and available at health food stores) contains hypericum and many other herbs useful in calming various conditions related to muscle spasm. It may take several weeks to see improvements from nutritional or herbal supplement programs. If your child is not making progress after about three months, see a naturopath or nutrition-oriented doctor for assessment of hidden food and chemical allergies, toxic heavy-metal excesses (especially of mercury), or candida overgrowth.

Post-Viral Muscle Problems

Muscle tension, spasm, pain, and the general aches after a viral illness have been termed post-viral neuromyasthenia. This can take months to clear but benefits from dietary changes and regular light exercise such as walking and stretching.

Dietary Recommendations

The most important dietary change is to eat more magnesium-rich foods, such as green vegetables. Following a high-alkaline-forming diet (high in fresh fruits and vegetables) helps prevent the loss of calcium, magnesium, potassium, and other vital muscle nutrients.

Avoid acid-forming foods:

> all animal foods, especially red meats and liver
>
> caffeinated beverages
>
> colas and soft drinks
>
> excessive amounts of grains
>
> highly processed foods high in phosphates
>
> refined sugars

Increase intake of alkaline-forming foods:

alfalfa

beets

brewer's yeast

carrots

cornmeal

fruits (especially apricots)

honey

leafy green vegetables (spinach, kale, lettuce, broccoli, celery, cucumber, sprouts)

millet

sesame seeds, pumpkin seeds

yogurt, kefir

Consider taking natural food supplements:

aloe vera juice

calcium

chlorophyll (best sources include barley green, blue-green algae, spirulina, and chlorella)

cramp bark herb tea

lobelia herb tea

magnesium

multimineral formula using colloidal minerals

potassium

silicon

vitamin B complex with extra niacin or niacinamide (B-3) and thiamin (B-1)

vitamin C

vitamin E

Topical Applications

Apply a mixture of equal parts evening primrose oil, olive oil, sesame seed oil or flaxseed oil, ginger juice, vitamin A, and zinc oxide several times daily until the muscle discomfort ceases. Hot packs, hot baths, and local Epsom salts packs (magnesium sulfate) are also effective in many cases. One can also put Epsom salts into bath water and soak in it daily until the pain and discomfort decrease. Tea tree oil in lotion or cream form can be applied before and after exercise to prevent or reduce symptom severity.

In more severe cases which respond poorly to this natural approach, I suggest magnesium sulfate injections (1,000 mg or more injected intramuscularly or intravenously two or three times weekly).

Prevention

Regular stretching prior to exercise and warm Epsom salts baths before bedtime can prevent muscle soreness, stiffness, and even cramps. Also, consider periodic visits for massage therapy, shiatsu, or chiropractic treatment.

Autism

Autism is a behavioral syndrome involving many causative factors and variously referred to as infantile autism, childhood autism, autistic disorder, pervasive developmental disorder, and childhood psychosis. The basic criteria for the presence of autism are some combinations of the following:

- Early onset (before three to five years of age)
- Severe abnormality in socially relating to others
- Severe abnormality of communication development (including language)
- Restricted, repetitive, and stereotyped patterns of behavior, interests, activities, and imagination
- Abnormal responses to sensory stimuli
- Marked lack of awareness of the existence of feelings of others
- Absence of or abnormal seeking of comfort at times of distress
- Absence of or impaired imitation
- Absence of or abnormal social play
- Impairment in making peer relationships
- No mode of communication such as communicative babbling, facial expression, gesture, mime, or spoken language
- Abnormal nonverbal communication with eye-to-eye gaze, facial expressions, or body posture
- Absent imaginative activity such as play-acting
- Abnormalities in speech production: volume, pitch, stress, rate, rhythm, and intonation
- Impairment in ability to initiate or sustain a conversation with others
- Stereotyped body movements: hand flicking, twisting, spinning, head banging
- Persistent preoccupation with parts of objects
- Marked distress with changes in trivial aspects of environment
- Unreasonable insistence on following routines in precise detail

- Markedly restricted range of interests and a preoccupation with one narrow interest

No one knows exactly what causes autism, but it is believed that a combination of several factors might be involved. Some of the many theories are that autism is a syndrome linked to:

amino acid imbalances or deficiencies

autoimmune mechanisms

candidiasis and parasitic disease

congenital or genetic defects

environmental or chemical effects

food allergies

intestinal malabsorption

leaky gut syndrome

psychological problems

toxic heavy-metal reactions

vaccinations

viruses

vitamin, mineral, and essential fatty acid deficiencies

The basic neurochemical process is thought to be related to abnormal dopamine metabolism or other neurotransmitter imbalances.

Many therapies have been claimed as helpful to autistic children including:

5-hydroxytryptophan or tryptophan

amino acid therapy

auditory integrative therapy

behavior therapy

bioflavonoids

chelation therapy for heavy-metal toxicity

choline

coenzyme Q10

detection and treatment of food and chemical allergies

DMG (dimethyl-glycine)

folic acid supplementation (particularly in autistic males with the fragile X syndrome)

ginkgo biloba extract

glutamine

intravenous gamma globulin

magnesium

octacosanol

other B complex vitamins

phenylalanine

treatment of candidiasis and parasites

treatment of hypothyroidism

tyrosine

vitamin B-5 (pantothenic acid)

vitamin B-6

vitamin C

vitamin E

Many autistic children suffer from hidden or delayed food allergies, especially to dairy and gluten products. Several published case reports indicate that nearly fifty percent of autistic cases improve when sugar, milk, and wheat are removed from the diet. Candidiasis and other chronic infections, especially parasites, are also commonly reported.

Gluten is the name of the protein found in the members of the grass family (wheat, oats, barley, kamut, quinoa, amaranth, spelt, rye, and triticale) and their derivatives (malt, grain starches, hydrolyzed vegetable/plant proteins, textured vegetable proteins, grain vinegars, soy sauce, grain alcohols, flavorings, and the binders and fillers found in many vitamins and medications). Casein is the name of the most common protein found in cow's milk, and it has a molecular structure nearly identical to that of gluten.

In the 1980s, Dr. C. Gillberg of London, England, produced evidence of elevated levels of "endorphin-like substances" (opioids or narcotic-like substances) in the cerebrospinal fluid of some children with autism, especially in those children who appeared to feel pain less than the normal population and who exhibited self-injurious behavior. There are abnormally elevated levels of similar opioids in the urine of about fifty percent of children with autism. Researchers have concluded that the quantities are such that they can only have been derived from the incomplete breakdown of certain foods.

Casein (from human or cow's milk) will break down in the stomach to produce a peptide known as casomorphine, which, as the name implies, will have opioid activities. Similar effects are noted with gluten from wheat and some other cereals such as oats, barley, and rye, which break down into opioid compounds called gluteomorphins or gliadinomorphins.

These biochemical facts are used as a rationale for treating autistic children with a diet that excludes casein from dairy products and gluten from grains. In general, children whose autism appears at or around the time of birth may have a problem with casein, whereas those whose autism becomes apparent at about two years of age are more likely to be reacting adversely to gluten. Some children may have difficulty with both since the molecules are so similar to each other, especially when it comes to their partially digested amino acid sequences. For an example of a dairy-free, gluten-free diet, see Appendix II.

Although there have been no attempts to demonstrate the effectiveness of such diets on a scientific basis, a significant number of parents have reported success in reversing autistic behavior by using the casein and/or gluten elimination diet.

Removal of gluten- and/or casein-containing products requires a great deal of discipline as well as the compliance and support of all those involved with the child's well-being. A well-meaning relative who ignores parental instruction and gives the child a glass of milk "because milk is the perfect food" can sabotage the treatment. In a similar way, a school teacher or psychotherapist who feels that the diet is nonsense and allows the child to eat junk food can lead parents to assume that the dairy-free, gluten-free diet is ineffective.

When the autistic child starts the gluten/casein-free diet, there may initially be withdrawal reactions such as upset stomach, anxiety, clinginess, and temper tantrums. These are, in reality, good signs; they will gradually change over a period of three months, eventually resulting in the reversal of some or a large percentage of the signs and symptoms of autism. If the response to the diet is positive, it should ideally be followed for about a year. If the diet does not work within three months, it is unlikely to do so if followed for any longer.

The adequacy of supplement dosages should be determined by objective testing through blood, urine, hair, and stool analysis. For magnesium, the red or white blood cell magnesium levels, twenty-four-hour urinary magnesium levels, and hair magnesium levels could be considered before deciding on dosages. Biochemical imbalances, infections, and functional problems could explain some common physical symptoms of autism such as constipation and chronic low mineral levels. Some of these causes are revealed by the following tests:

- CDSA and CP (comprehensive digestive and stool analysis with comprehensive parasitology): these tests have their main value in the assessment of how well a person digests and assimilates his or her food and whether there is bacterial bowel flora imbalance, hidden infection with yeast or parasites, food allergy, low stomach acidity, or digestive enzyme insufficiency. Children who fail to gain weight on even high-calorie, healthy diets may be lacking sufficient hydrochloric acid in their stomach or have a low output of digestive enzymes from their pancreas. Once the specific functional problem is determined by the CDSA, further investigation and treatment can be carried out as indicated by the results of the test.

- Live-cell microscopy: this is not a diagnostic procedure for any specific disease; it is best used as a screening test to help determine the optimal diet and natural therapies for a given individual with chronic illness, especially of the immune system. Analysis of the blood by the microscope is as old as the practice of medicine itself. The main advantage of blood microscopy is that many nutritional imbalances can be detected before standard chemical blood tests show any abnormalities. Health problems can then be prevented by early nutritional intervention. (See Chapter 2 for more information.)

- Food and chemical allergy testing: a variety of tests that can reveal hidden or delayed allergies. In the past decade of my practice, I have been using the elimination-provocation test when appropriate, combined with the ELISA/Act test. In my opinion and experience, this combination represents the state of the art in detecting hidden food sensitivities. The scientific literature certainly supports this approach.

Attention Deficit Disorder

Attention deficit disorder (ADD) affects thousands of infants, children, adolescents, and adults. It shows up as abnormalities in behavior such as hyperactivity, learning disorders, and communication problems in early childhood, with remission sometimes occurring during puberty. The remission may or may not last depending on individual circumstances. It is thought that children are usually affected by ADD before birth and, left untreated, continue to suffer from the condition into adulthood. ADD affects more boys than girls, at a ratio of 3:1. A high percentage of hyperactive children have blond hair and blue eyes and suffer from what appear to be allergic signs and symptoms.

In the history of an ADD child, the mother often recalls that, during pregnancy, there was a great deal of fetal movement and very hard kicking. As infants, hyperactive babies are often colicky, sleep poorly or very little, and cry or scream a lot. In childhood, they look restless and fidgety and eat poorly. In the more severe cases, they may be "rockers" or "head bangers," rejecting affection and mothering.

As ADD children become older, they have short attention spans, are easily distracted, and rush from one thing to the next. Behavior can become destructive, with poor coordination and general clumsiness. Some hyperactive children have trouble integrating what they see and hear due to visual perception abnormalities which, in turn, lead to an inability to understand basic concepts.

Other conditions that occur in many ADD children include eczema, asthma, chronic infections, hay fever, headaches, stomachaches, and fungal infections of the scalp, skin, and nails.

Symptoms of ADD in infants and young children:

crying inconsolably

difficult feeding

fits or temper tantrums

head banging or rocking

poor or little sleep

rejection of affection and cuddling

restlessness

screaming

Symptoms of ADD in older children:

accident-proneness

aggressiveness

bed-wetting (enuresis)

bouts of fatigue, weakness, and listlessness

clumsiness

constantly moving

dark circles or puffiness below the eyes

destructive or disruptive behavior

hypersensitivity to odors, lights, sound, heat, and cold

impulsiveness

irritability, disobedience, lack of cooperation, self-injurious behavior

nervousness, moodiness, or depression

nose and skin picking or hair pulling

poor appetite and erratic eating habits

poor concentration ability

poor coordination

poor sleep, nightmares

red earlobes or red cheeks

restlessness

school failure despite normal or high IQ

swollen neck glands or fluid behind eardrums

vocal repetition and loudness

withdrawn behavior

Causes of ADD:

- biochemical imbalances caused by toxic heavy metals (lead or cadmium excesses), food allergies, vitamin and mineral deficiencies, amino acid deficiencies
- birth injuries
- digestive enzyme or stomach acid deficiencies
- dyes, chemicals, inhalants, and other irritants
- environmental hypersensitivities, especially to food dyes, chemicals, and additives
- genetic abnormalities
- hormonal imbalances
- hypoglycemia or sugar hypersensitivity
- multiple food cravings and delayed (type II–IV) allergies
- psychological or emotional problems
- toxins from chronic infections with bacteria, fungi, and parasites

ADD children should be thoroughly tested and treated by diet changes and nutritional supplements before resorting to amphetamine-like drugs such as methylphenidate.

Tests to consider:

- amino acid analysis
- CDSA and comprehensive parasitology
- ELISA/Act blood test
- food and chemical allergy testing
- gut-permeability testing
- hair mineral analysis

- hormonal tests for thyroid, adrenal, pancreas (enzymes, insulin, glucagon)
- insulin and glucose tolerance tests
- live-cell microscopy
- routine blood and urine tests
- vitamin and mineral testing

Nutritional Deficiencies and ADD

Micronutrient deficiencies (e.g., zinc) or dependencies on high levels of zinc supplementation in order to behave normally can have deleterious effects on both short- and long-term memory. White spots on the nails could be a sign of zinc deficiency even when blood tests for zinc are normal. The expression "No zinc, no think" is not without merit. Many studies have shown that zinc supplementation is helpful with memory, thinking, and IQ. The best way of getting zinc is to optimize the diet. The most recently published RDA (recommended dietary allowance) for children is 15 mg per day. The richest sources of zinc are generally the high-protein foods such as organ meats, seafood (especially shellfish), whole grains, and legumes (beans and peas).

Cognitive impairment may also be associated with a deficiency in iron. Studies show that cognitive development can be impaired when there are low blood iron levels. Deficiencies in B-vitamins, particularly vitamin B-1 and choline may also be involved.

The Role of Heavy Metals and Amino Acids

Toxic heavy metals such as cadmium and lead can accumulate in the body and cause both hyperactive behavior and learning disabilities in some susceptible children. A hair mineral analysis can indicate whether these toxic heavy metals are building up in the body. The good news is that, with a natural program of vitamins and minerals, accumulations of lead and cadmium can be removed from the system.

Since amino acids are the precursors to the neurotransmitters, low levels can lead to neurotransmitter deficiency. Higher than accepted levels may lead to neurotransmitter excess. One example of amino acid excess causing hyperactive behavior occurs with the artificial sweetener aspartame. Some children are highly sensitive to aspartame, and scrupulous attention should be aimed at keeping this potential neurotoxin out of the sensitive child's diet. Amino acid levels can be significantly abnormal in children who consume large amounts of aspartame in soft drinks or other processed foods. Once the amino acid levels are determined, treatment can be aimed at balancing brain chemicals more accurately.

The Use of Amphetamine-Like Drugs

Practitioners of conventional medicine treat ADD children with amphetamine-like drugs. These stimulant medications work fairly quickly, and this is effective treatment for many children—especially in the case of the child about to be expelled from school or causing the family to fall apart. Other positive factors are that these drugs are relatively inexpensive, are easy to administer, and can be used safely for many years. Recent studies have shown that amphetamine-like drugs in huge doses can cause cancer in lab mice, but there is no evidence that this occurs in children.

On the negative side, amphetamine-like drugs are only effective in about seventy to seventy-five percent of cases. In many cases, increased hyperactivity occurs after the last dose of the day has worn off. The child may experience a loss of appetite and have trouble going to sleep and getting up in the morning. The risk of marginal deficiencies in iron, zinc, calcium, B vitamins, protein, and so on increases with the loss of appetite.

Amphetamine-like drugs do not address the cause of ADD/hyperactivity. It's akin to taking an aspirin for recurrent headaches: the pain goes away temporarily, but the reasons for the headaches remain unaddressed. The majority of parents do not like the idea of medicating their children. Some parents reluctantly medicate their children only because they are pressured by teachers, schools, and dogmatic physicians to use stimulant drugs. Furthermore, there are no long-term studies showing that medicated children do better in the long run academically, emotionally, or otherwise compared to the children of parents who say "no" to drugs.

Natural Treatments for ADD

Aside from dietary changes to eliminate sugar, caffeine, and food and chemical allergens, there are many natural treatments for ADD, including a long list of vitamins, minerals, herbs, amino acids, essential fatty acids, and enzymes. Highly effective natural supplements for ADD:

Vitamins, minerals, and antioxidants:

> vitamin A, beta carotene
>
> B complex vitamin
>
> vitamin C
>
> pycnogenol
>
> quercetin
>
> coenzyme Q10
>
> vitamin E
>
> calcium
>
> chromium
>
> iron
>
> magnesium
>
> manganese
>
> vanadyl sulfate
>
> zinc

Amino acids:

> arginine
>
> GABA (gamma amino butyric acid)
>
> glutamine
>
> ornithine
>
> D- , L-phenylalanine
>
> tryptophan
>
> tyrosine

Essential fatty acids:

> black currant oil
>
> borage oil
>
> evening primrose oil
>
> flaxseed oil
>
> olive oil
>
> salmon oil

Digestive enzymes:

> betaine and pepsin
>
> glutamic acid
>
> pancreatin
>
> plant enzymes
>
> probiotics (*lactobacillus, acidophilus*)

Herbs:

> burdock
>
> chamomile
>
> garlic
>
> *Ginkgo biloba* extract

gotu cola

gymnema

hypericum (St. John's wort)

ma huang

Siberian ginseng

taheebo

valerian

A hypoallergenic or rotation diet may also help. The appropriate treatment depends on the case history, physical examination, and the results of biochemical tests.

Evening primrose oil is a common remedy recommended for ADD children and, together with other aspects of a comprehensive biochemical treatment program, can be helpful in reversing the disorder. Primrose oil and herbs such as licorice root, curcumin, and alfalfa have anti-inflammatory and anti-allergy properties through the ability to modulate levels of prostaglandin—the hormones responsible for inflammation, pain, allergic reactions, and other aspects of the immune system.

Based on the findings of biochemical tests, a personalized nutritional program of diet and supplements can be recommended. Work with a naturopath or a medical doctor familiar with nutritional remedies.

Learning Disabilities

A learning disability (LD) is defined as a disorder in one or more of the basic psychological processes involved in understanding which results in an imperfect ability to listen, think, speak, read, write, or spell.

Characteristics of a child with a learning disability include:

• difficulty distinguishing among letters, numbers, and sounds

• difficulty naming familiar things or people

- difficulty telling time or right from left
- difficulty understanding words or concepts
- difficulty with sounding out words
- discipline problems
- impulsiveness
- inability to follow directions
- inappropriate responses
- late gross or fine motor development
- late speech development
- poor coordination
- poor listening skills
- poor memory
- poor reading and writing
- restlessness
- reversing letters
- short attention span

Like the other chronic diseases of our times—multiple sclerosis (MS), lupus, cancer, CFS, asthma, and autoimmune disease—LD is at epidemic levels in the post industrial–revolution era. Childhood learning problems are definitely on the rise. Some argue that this is because of better recognition and objective testing, but respected authors such as William Crook, M.D., and Lendon Smith, M.D., strongly disagree.

Learning disability was not a major problem for children growing up in the early 1800s. As recently as 1950, there was only one child in each classroom with LD; today, that number is more like five or six. Amphetamine-like drugs and intense psychotherapy have done nothing to slow the dramatic rise in the incidence of this diagnosis because they do not address the source of the problem. The answers to why a child develops LD lie in the fields of genetics, environmental toxicology, and nutrition.

Although genetics, infections, and brain damage (trauma) have been cited as causes of LD, these cases are quite rare compared to causes such as a dysfunctional home, heavy-metal toxicities, nutritional deficiencies, and food and chemical allergies. The majority of cases are caused by an immune defect and allergies to food additives, preservatives, chemicals, or inhalants. To deal adequately with this illness, we must address all these potential imbalances. Some of the nutritional deficiencies that correlate with LD are calcium, magnesium, iodine, iron, and zinc. On the other hand, high copper, lead, cadmium, and aluminum levels have also been seen in learning-disabled children.

Allergies and LD

An allergy may make a student tired, listless, nauseated, and even irritable. The majority of conventional doctors, however, dismiss allergies as the cause of learning disabilities and school problems. They believe that both absenteeism and learning disabilities are preventable with proper medication, supportive environmental controls, attention to coping strategies, and family education. Studies published by authors such as William Crook have been dismissed by conventional doctors as "anecdotal." Anecdotal or not, parents find it hard to ignore the fact that their child recovers from a learning disability when milk and wheat are removed from the diet.

Allergies have been implicated in case studies of specific learning disabilities and associated with lower performance in reading, auditory perception, and visual perception. Teacher and parent ratings, as well as test scores, have indicated lower proficiency among allergic students. Students with LD who have recurrent otitis media have also been found to have more problems with allergies and verbal skills than nondisabled children. Children with asthma and chronic rhinitis tended to be rated lower in listening skills, and hearing difficulties have been associated with otitis media resulting from allergies.

A history of problems connected to allergies has also been reported for behavioral problems such as being overtalkative, irritable, inattentive/distractible, hyperactive, impulsive, difficult to handle, drowsy/sleepy, mean, withdrawn, and euphoric. Hyperactivity has been particularly connected with food allergies, chemical allergies, and salicylate sensitivity.

Problems with allergy medications: Certain allergy medications have been reported to have adverse side effects on learning and behavior because they affect the central nervous system. For example, the use of the antiasthma drug theophylline has been significantly correlated with reports of inattentiveness, hyperactivity, irritability, drowsiness, and withdrawal behavior; these negative side effects are directly proportional to the length of use. The use of this medication may also cause learning disabilities.

Corticosteroids are other drugs used to treat asthma, allergic rhinitis, and other allergic conditions. Unfortunately, these drugs have both direct and indirect impacts on the central nervous system. They have been documented to cause mood changes, changes in brain electrical activity, changes in sleep patterns, increased irritability, and even psychotic reactions. Children continuously on steroids for at least a year have been reported to have lower performance on standardized academic achievement tests for reading, verbal memory, and mathematics.

Commonly used prescription and over-the-counter antihistamines have been reported to cause drowsiness, slower reaction times on visual-motor tasks, and worsened attention and cerebral processing speed. Antihistamines can also cause sedation, dry mouth, and irritability. In some children, decongestants have been associated with visual hallucinations. While spokespersons for the medical profession tend to minimize such side effects, they can be of significant concern to parents of children with learning disabilities.

There are many nautral alternatives to antihistamines, decongestants, and steroids. The following supplements can help offset symptoms and enhance immunity:

- vitamin A
- beta-carotene
- B complex vitamins (especially B-5 and B-6)
- vitamin C
- vitamin E
- germanium
- selenium
- zinc
- coenzyme Q10
- bioflavonoids
- glutathione
- aloe vera juice
- bee pollen
- spirulina and other green drinks
- N-acetyl-cysteine
- colloidal silver
- essential fatty acids
- calcium, magnesium, and potassium bicarbonate mixture
- curcumin (from cumin)
- betaine, pepsin
- all plant and pancreatic digestive enzymes
- echinacea
- goldenseal
- hypericum
- lomatium
- astragalus
- calendula

- gentian
- *ma huang*
- peppermint oil
- *salix alba*
- tea tree oil
- taheebo
- garlic
- capsicum
- horehound
- licorice root
- elderberry
- red clover

Childhood Depression

Childhood depression is not always caused by psychiatric or psychological conflicts. It is more often related to an excessive consumption of sucrose (sugar) and deficiencies of biotin, folic acid, other B complex vitamins, vitamin C, zinc, calcium, copper, iron, magnesium, or potassium. Depression can also be caused by excesses of magnesium or vanadium, by imbalances in amino acids, and by food allergies.

There is a definite benefit to be gained by giving vitamin B-12 to depressed children. The effective therapeutic dose of vitamin B-12 is highly variable, but a trial therapy of 3,000 mcg taken daily under the tongue (sublingual) or as a nasal gel may be effective after two or three weeks. If not, daily, weekly, or monthly intramuscular injections may be worth a try until symptoms resolve.

Other effective nutritional antidepressants include lithium, phenylalanine, tyrosine, tryptophan, melatonin, and hypericum (from St. John's wort).

The Role of Serotonin and Tryptophan

Serotonin is a very important brain biochemical and must be present at optimal levels to prevent depression. One natural way of increasing its level in the brain is to take tryptophan, the amino acid precursor of serotonin. Tryptophan is an essential amino acid found in high amounts in fish, meat, dairy products, eggs, nuts, and wheat germ. It is also found in lesser amounts in the herb chamomile, long recognized for its soothing effects. Children who have trouble digesting high-protein foods may not be getting the tryptophan they need from their diets. As a result, brain serotonin levels may get low and lead to depression, obsessive-compulsive disorders, mania, anxiety, insomnia, eating disorders, and obesity. Tryptophan is available through health care practitioners in the United States. In Canada, it is available by prescription from any general practitioner.

It's best to get a plasma amino acid analysis done before taking high-dose supplements of any amino acid. Tryptophan is made more effective by also taking vitamins B-3 (niacinamide), B-6, and C. Its uptake in the brain is enhanced by taking it with a high-carbohydrate meal (e.g., pasta, fruit, vegetables, or starches). Foods which contain preformed serotonin also increase brain uptake of tryptophan. These foods include bananas, walnuts, and pineapples.

Food allergies, candida infection, parasites, and toxic heavy metals may all have deleterious effects on digestion and hence on tryptophan absorption or utilization. If digestion is poor, supplemental betaine and pepsin, glutamic acid, apple cider vinegar, Swedish bitters, pancreatin, plant enzymes, *lactobacillus acidophilus,* or other digestive aids may need to be used. A naturopath or holistic doctor can order tests such as a CDSA (comprehensive digestive and stool analysis) or live-cell microscopy to diagnose possible maldigestion. Specific therapy could then be instituted to optimize the digestive system.

Asthma

Asthma is a hypersensitivity condition of the lungs resulting in coughing, wheezing, breathing difficulties, and production of bronchial mucus. Asthma is the major cause of school absenteeism for children under fifteen years of age in the United States and can be a life-threatening condition. It is especially severe in children between the ages of ten and fifteen years old.

Asthma results from a constriction of smooth muscles which line the tiny airways of the lungs. Inflammation is caused by chronic infection, chemical exposure, or allergens. Certain herbs and nutrients can help the muscles relax and permit the airways to open.

Facts about asthma:

- Asthma affects approximately five percent of the population (fifteen million Americans), of which fifty percent are children.

- Asthma occurs most commonly in children under the age of ten, with 2:1 male-to-female ratio.

- There has been an eighty-percent increase in the prevalence and incidence of asthma since 1980; air pollution, increasing levels of chemicals in children's diets, and the weakening of the immune system by antibiotics are often cited as causes.

- Increasing asthma rates parallel the increased presence of chemicalized household products, scents, wood preservatives, floor and wall treatments, carpets, rugs, drapes, and synthetic-impregnated furniture.

- Increasing asthma rates also coincide with a relative increase in indoor house mite infestation and indoor natural gas (from furnaces, water heaters, and stoves), which generates irritative nitric oxide residues.

- Since 1980, the mortality rate from asthma has increased three hundred percent in total, and two hundred percent in children.

- There is a two hundred-percent increase in the risk of death due to asthma in African American children compared to white children.

  There are basically two types of asthma:

1. Extrinsic/atopic ("allergic") asthma is mediated by the IgE family of allergens: dust, molds, pollens, animal danders, tobacco smoke and foods. Exposure results in an immediate allergic reaction.
2. Intrinsic asthma is mediated through cold air, exercise, infection, emotional upset, and other irritants.

  Most children have a mixture of the two types, with the allergic (extrinsic) type being more common. Asthma prescription sprays and pills provide temporary relief but do nothing to halt the progression of the disease and may actually hasten it. There is growing evidence that the commonly used adrenaline-like bronchodilators profoundly increase or worsen asthma.

  Childhood asthma can best be treated by using a combination of conventional and natural therapies as needed. The natural approaches are most applicable in the prevention of wheezing attacks and associated infections. Conventional medicine uses synthetic corticosteroids to suppress inflammation, but parents should be aware of natural alternatives.

Natural Anti-Inflammatory Supplements

- Chinese skullcap (*Scutellaria baicalensis*): anti-inflammatory, high in flavonoids
- Curcumin, the yellow pigment of turmeric (*Curcuma longa*): primarily an anti-inflammatory agent, comparable to cortisone, ibuprofen, and phenylbutazone
- Essential fatty acids (evening primrose oil, flaxseed oil, borage oil, black currant seed oil)
- Forskolin (a derivative of the herb *Coleus forskoli*): found to be a good natural bronchodilator. It does this by inhibiting the

release of pro-inflammatory compounds and inhibiting the smooth muscle contraction in the airways. Forskolin reduces inflammatory reactions thought to contribute to asthma without systemic side effects.

- Ephedra (*ma huang*) has been used for over five thousand years in Chinese medicine; anti-inflammatory and antiallergenic ephedrine component. Its effect diminishes unless used in combination with other herbs for adrenal support (licorice root, ginseng, vitamin C, magnesium, zinc, vitamin B-6, and pantothenic acid).

- Licorice (*glycyrrhiza glabra*): anti-inflammatory and antiallergenic action due to ability to increase half-life of cortisol

- Magnesium (relaxes bronchial smooth muscle)

- Selenium (reduces leukotriene formation)

- Vitamin B-12 (Dr. Jonathan Wright has shown that 1 mg or more injected weekly is effective in reversing asthma)

- Vitamin B-6

- Vitamin C (asthmatics have been shown to have lower serum and white cell ascorbic acid levels)

- Vitamin E

- *Ginkgo biloba*

- Carotenes

- Glutathione

- Coenzyme Q10

Natural Dietary Treatments for Asthma

- For symptomatic relief, give the child plenty of distilled or reverse-osmosis water to loosen bronchial secretions.

- For longer-term therapy change the diet from animal-based to more plant-based foods. One study showed a ninety-two-percent improvement in asthmatic patients when all animal products were eliminated from their diet. This vegan diet is successful because it eliminates common food allergens and alters fatty-acid metabolism, which reduces the production of pro-inflammatory leukotrienes. Leukotrienes are also pro-allergenic, because these come from arachidonic acid—a fatty acid found exclusively in animal products.

- Irrespective of food or other allergies, asthmatics should avoid sugar and white flour products because of their negative effects on the immune system.

- Children with asthma have been shown to have a defect in tryptophan metabolism. Double-blind studies show benefits from a tryptophan-restricted diet. Restricting tryptophan prevents a reaction due to the fact that is is poorly broken down. If tryptophan is restricted, it does not accumulate and cause problems. Vitamin B-6 supplementation can also help to correct tryptophan metabolism, thereby lessening asthmatic symptoms.

- Identify food and chemical allergies by skin tests for immediate allergies, elimination-provocation techniques, and/or blood tests. Common immediate allergens are eggs, fish, shellfish, nuts, and peanuts; common delayed allergens include milk, chocolate, wheat, citrus, and food colorings.

- It has been known for over sixty years that most asthmatics produce too little hydrochloric acid in their stomachs. In 1931, G. W. Bray published an article entitled "The Hypochlorhydria of Asthma of Childhood" in the *Quarterly Journal of Medicine*. The article showed that eighty percent of asthmatics had stomach acid levels below normal and that asthma can be alleviated by supplementing acid intake (with glutamic acid, betaine and pepsin, stomach bitters, or other digestive enzyme supplements).

- Many asthmatics have poor pancreatic function and inadequate secretion of digestive enzymes. As a result, high-protein foods may not be digested completely and, when absorbed into the bloodstream, may evoke an allergic reaction such as wheezing. Supplementation with pancreatic digestive enzymes or plant enzymes halps break down high-protein foods to their individual amino acids, which are nonallergenic. Asthma attacks are thus prevented.

- Eliminate food additives: dyes such as tartrazine which are likely to be found in processed foods, drugs, canned foods, soft drinks, and most junk food, preservatives such as sodium benzoate, sulfur dioxide and other sulfites (e.g., metabisulfite), and anything containing aspartame. Sulfites, used as a preservative in many foods and beverages, can precipitate asthma. Learn to become a label reader and avoid all these known asthma triggers. In restaurants, the problem may be much more difficult since sulfites are used liberally in practically all dishes, especially salads. Commonly used sulfites include sodium bisulfite, potassium metabisulfite, potassium bisulfite, and sulfur dioxide. Test strips are now available to detect the presence of sulfites in foods (write to: Sulfitest, Center Laboratories, 35 Channel Dr., Port Washington, NY 11050 or call 516-767-1800).

- Sensitivity to aspirin and NSAIDs (nonsteroidal anti-inflammatory drugs) can induce asthma attacks in sensitive individuals via the excessive release of inflammatory chemicals from mast cells. Many children are sensitive to salicylates, which are found in aspirin and in many natural foods. These items should be eliminated from the diet if the asthmatic is sensitive to salicylates. (See Appendix II.)

Physical Treatments for Asthma

- Use a vaporizer with eucalyptus or thyme leaves added to the water.
- Breathing exercises and yoga have been proven to reverse symptoms of asthma in selected individuals.
- Massage therapy, acupuncture, acupressure/shiatsu, chiropractic, and osteopathic treatments may all help.

Additional Supplements for the Treatment of Asthma

- *Angelica sinensis:* antiallergenic; prevents production of IgE antibodies
- Astragalus: an herb that boosts immunity and lung strength
- Bioflavonoids (quercetin, proanthocyanidins, hesperidin, catechin, rutin): powerful antioxidants that help stabilize the mast cell membrane and strengthen capillaries and other blood vessels by not allowing easy histamine release or excessive inflammation to occur.
- Capsicum (chili pepper): capsaicin, the major active component, desensitizes airways, improves circulation, and kills unfriendly microbes in the gastrointestinal tract
- Echinacea: natural antibiotic herb
- Elecampane: effective herbal cough remedy; has antimicrobial properties
- Garlic and onions: high in vitamin C and quercetin (bioflavonoid); inhibit production of leukotrienes
- Green tea: helps open airways due to its theophylline content and antioxidants
- Herbal expectorants: lobelia, licorice root, grindelia, euphorbia, sundew, and senega
- Iodine: in the form of SSKI (saturated solution of potassium iodide) or Lugol's solution is effective as an expectorant in cases of asthma and bronchitis complicated by mucus congestion
- *Lactobacillus acidophilus* and bifidobacteria (dairy-free): help prevent colonization of the gastrointestinal tract with unfriendly/pathogenic microbes such as candida and parasites
- Lobelia: expectorant; releases adrenal hormones, helping to relax bronchial muscles
- Mullein: antispasmodic, decongestant
- N-acetyl-cysteine: mucolytic natural antibiotic; stimulates the production of glutathione—a powerful antioxidant—in the body
- Thyme: antispasmodic

Childhood Diabetes

Childhood diabetes (juvenile or insulin-dependent diabetes mellitus, or IDDM) has been shown to result from an autoimmune disease mechanism. Evidence continues to mount that one of the triggers of IDDM is an allergy to cow's milk albumin and possibly to wheat gliadin, a protein found in wheat. IDDM affects nearly two million children and young adults in North America. It is responsible for over twenty-five thousand amputations and at least thirty-seven thousand deaths each year. In addition to eliminating simple sugars from the diet, a wise preventive action would be to test children for antibodies in their blood against cow's milk and wheat.

There is effective complementary medical therapy for childhood diabetes. Although many of the self-help nutritional and herbal supplements are without significant side effects, drug interactions are possible in children who are taking oral hypoglycemic drugs or insulin injections. Ideally, work with a sympathetic medical doctor to supervise progress. If a child is taking any amount of insulin or hypoglycemic drugs, make sure you monitor the blood sugar levels with a glucometer at least twice a day or as directed by your health care practitioner.

Eating Plan

- Eliminate sugar in any amount. Sugar increases the body's loss of chromium through the urine and leads directly to glucose intolerance (i.e., diabetes and hypoglycemia). Sugar in moderation is unrealistic for any diabetic; it is hazardous and perpetuates the disease. Sugar depresses the immune system and acts as an appetite stimulant; the more sugar one eats, the more one is likely to eat in general.
- Feed your child an HCF (high complex carbohydrate, high fiber) diet: seventy percent of calories from complex carbohydrates, fifteen percent from protein, fifteen percent from fat. The closer the diet is to vegetarian principles the better.

Include one to two servings of fruit daily, depending on blood sugar response.

• Give five to six small meals throughout the day instead of large meals.

• Ideally, use a hypoallergenic/rotation diet (see Appendix II). If at all possible, have food allergy testing done by your doctor using the ELISA blood test; eliminate the allergenic foods and place everything else on a four-day rotation. This is especially important to the overweight diabetic.

Foods to emphasize: Chromium is an essential mineral and is an active ingredient in a substance called GTF (glucose tolerance factor), along with vitamin B-3 (niacin) and amino acids. Of the supplements, chromium picolinate is the best absorbed and utilized by the body.

Feed your child more of the following blood sugar–controlling foods (provided no allergies exist to them):

Chromium-rich foods:

brewer's yeast, whole grains, mushrooms, beets, grapes, raisins, cucumber, garlic, Jerusalem artichokes, parsley, string beans

Zinc-rich foods:

sunflower and squash seeds, peanuts, meats, wheat germ, soy meal, hard wheat berries, wheat bran, buckwheat, rice bran, millet, whole wheat flour, oatmeal, brown rice, corn-meal, black-eyed peas, green beans, chickpeas, lima beans, spinach, green onions, green leafy vegetables, sprouted grains

Foods high in water-soluble fiber:

psyllium, flaxseed, pectin, guar gum, and bran

Complex whole-grain and legume carbohydrates:

pumpkin, whole rice, yams, mung beans, squash, celery, peach, millet, onion, spinach, blueberries, peas, tofu, cabbage, radish

Foods rich in other trace minerals such as iodine and silicon:

kelp, dulse, Swiss chard, turnip greens, sesame seeds, other seeds and nuts, raw goat's milk, garlic, wheat germ, liquid chlorophyll, alfalfa sprouts, buckwheat, watercress, rice polishings, apples, celery, cherries onions, beans, legumes, soy, ginger, alfalfa, yogurt, brewer's yeast

Omega-3 and omega-6 fatty acid–containing foods:

vegetable, nut, and seed oils; salmon, herring, mackerel, sardines, walnuts, flaxseed oil, evening primrose oil, black currant oil

Spices:

cinnamon, turmeric, bay leaf, cloves

Therapeutic fresh juices and teas:

huckleberry leaf tea; parsley tea; raw sauerkraut and lemon; raw sauerkraut and tomato; string bean, brussels sprouts, carrot, and lettuce; string bean, cucumber, and celery; watermelon and tomato

Foods to avoid:

- food allergens, fried foods, caffeine, spicy foods, processed foods
- sugars (glucose, fructose, lactose, malt, maltose, dextrose, corn syrup), candy, honey, molasses, dried fruits, concentrated sweets, concentrated juices
- trans-fatty acids from hydrogenated oils (margarine, vegetable shortenings, imitation butter spreads, most commercial peanut butters) and oxidized fats (deep-fried foods, fast food, ghee, barbecued meats)
- iron (diabetes has been found with increasing frequency in those with high blood levels of ferritin, or stored iron)

Recommended supplements: Doses should be determined by biochemical tests, individual needs, and practitioner supervision.

Several companies group these supplements in combination tablets or capsules, significantly reducing the number of pills to be taken. As improvement occurs, doses can be reduced and many of the supplements can be stopped.

• beta carotene

• bioflavonoids (pycnogenol, rutin, hesperidin, and quercetin)

• biotin

• burdock root (a plant source of insulin)

• cedar berries (a plant source of insulin)

• chromium picolinate

• coenzyme Q10

• copper citrate

• folic acid

• *Ginkgo biloba* extract (helps prevent diabetic retinopathy and peripheral vascular disease)

• goldenseal root

• *Gymnema sylvestre* (an herb that lowers the level of blood sugar)

• inulin (a fructo-oligosaccharide derived from dahlia, dandelion, or chicory; stabilizes blood sugar levels and helps increase the population of bifidobacteria in the intestines)

• L-carnitine

• licorice root

• magnesium

• manganese

• myoinositol (especially helpful in cases of neuropathy)

• niacin (vitamin B-3, time-release)

• omega-3 fatty acids and omega-6 fatty acids (flaxseed oil, salmon oil, evening primrose oil)

• potassium citrate

• selenium

- silica (horsetail)

- uva ursi

- vanadyl sulfate (produces an insulin-like reaction when taken with meals)

- vitamin B-1

- vitamin B-6

- vitamin B-12

- vitamin C (note: if ferritin or blood iron levels are high, vitamin C should not be supplemented in high doses until levels return to normal; vitamin C increases iron absorption and may worsen iron toxicity problems)

- vitamin E

- zinc picolinate

Alfalfa, aloe vera, garlic, onions, fenugreek, capsicum, ginger, kelp, liquid chlorophyll, blue-green algae, psyllium, ginseng, and *lactobacillus acidophilus* may all be used to provide other trace minerals and promote tissue healing, digestion, and elimination.

At first glance, all of this might seem overwhelming. The good news is that implementing only a few of the suggested changes can lower the requirements for insulin and hypoglycemic drugs dramatically. For example, several studies indicate that just increasing the fiber content of the diet to forty grams per day while eliminating refined sugars lowers insulin requirements by as much as thirty percent.

Nephrotic Syndrome

Nephrotic syndrome is characterized by excess protein in the urine, low albumin in the blood, high blood fats, and edema (fluid retention). There are many health conditions associated with nephrotic syndrome. Each case must be treated somewhat differently. Food allergy or intolerance may be the cause of some cases of nephrotic syndrome.

In serious medical conditions, homeopathic/naturopathic medicine can only be considered complementary to conventional medical treatment. In many cases, there are no alternatives to the medical approach, which involves the use of cortisone-like drugs. In some children, the natural approach is effective in reducing or eliminating the need for cortisone.

If a child is taking cortisone-like drugs, zinc supplementation may be needed. Cortisone and many other drugs tend to make the body lose zinc in greater amounts than can easily be obtained from the diet. This could then result in poor wound healing, hair loss, a failure to thrive, short body stature, and taste perception problems.

Children who are taking steroids should be given a twenty-four-hour urine test for minerals such as calcium, magnesium, phosphorus, copper, and zinc. Also, hair mineral analysis can be done to find out about excesses of toxic heavy metals in the body, such as cadmium, lead, mercury, aluminum, nickel, copper, and arsenic. Some of these metals can be stored in the body for long periods of time and lead to kidney damage.

8 Dealing Effectively with Conventional Doctors and Medical Politics

Examining the Conventional Doctor

The word "doctor" comes from the Latin *docere*, which means "to teach." Real doctors teach their patients about prevention, health, and healing. In the Hippocratic or classical view of healing, the responsibility for health lies with the patient, while the doctor is more of an educator. Unfortunately, this classical attitude is not taught in medical schools. Medical schools today teach the doctor-as-God model. This gives responsibility for health matters to the doctor—an approach that is attractive to the quick-fix mentality of many North Americans.

Medical schooling and the militaristic behavior of medical professionals, especially in hospitals, imprints an almost religious conviction on newly minted doctors. Most doctors believe what they are told to believe; this mentality leads to few innovations, a suspicion of anything unfamiliar, and institutionalized mediocrity. Throughout their careers doctors continue to believe, "If I didn't hear about it in medical school, it must not be any good."

Most doctors stay locked into this system, practicing medicine as it is endorsed by medical schools, the American Medical Association (AMA), the Food and Drug Administration (FDA), state medical boards, and other organizations such as the American Cancer Society (ACS) and the National Cancer Institute (NCI). Doctors influenced by these groups are seldom willing to consider the possibility that effective remedies could come from outside these institutions.

On the other hand, complementary medical practitioners (holistic doctors or alternative medicine doctors) are those who have had the self-determination to overcome medical school dogma and think for themselves. Complementary medical doctors see themselves mainly as teachers, not necessarily interveners. They focus on health as opposed to disease and employ primarily drugless means to help people prevent illness.

Why Most Doctors Avoid Alternative Medicine

Have you noticed that most visits to a family doctor or specialist are brief? The average office visit lasts eight minutes. This is because conventional doctors act as interveners who diagnose a disease or syndrome, prescribe FDA-approved drugs, and refer anyone with symptoms that fail to conform to recognized organic illness to see a psychiatrist.

Doctors behave this way often from a fear of lawsuits. Anything odd, different, or disapproved of by mainstream medical dogma is turned over to a specialist, most often a psychiatrist. Everything has to be justified by lab tests and treated by the book. The only treatments often offered are those that will be supported by the medical community in court, that will be acceptable to malpractice insurance companies, and that health insurance companies will cover. New or controversial treatments are sometimes regarded by mainstream doctors as professional suicide.

Doctors also fear a loss of income if they recommend natural remedies not covered by insurance companies. Every treatment must be justified according to insurance company guidelines. For all practical purposes, neither patient nor doctor has any control over what is allowed or not allowed by insurance companies. This prevents doctors from ordering any special nutritional medical testing, most of which are not covered by insurance companies.

Malpractice insurance and the other costs that lead to high office overhead leave little profit for the average private practitioner, so the name of the game becomes "see as many patients as you can." There is no time for listening to patients' opinions; talk-intensive alternative medicine, with its emphasis on education, is just bad business. The object becomes to cure the symptom as quickly as possible and keep the patient from complaining. To this end, doctors will use the drug that requires the least time and causes the fewest side effects to the doctor, not the patient.

Although many conventional doctors are aware that most disease and injury result from behavior and diet, they are also convinced that people will not change their diets and lifestyles to exclude bad habits such as sugar or high fat intake. The average doctor shrugs, "Why bother telling patients to change?" Conventional doctors continue to treat patients with available drugs for a quick fix and avoid the risk of beating their heads against a brick wall with detailed advice on diet and lifestyle changes. In essence, today's doctor has become a businessperson first, a lawyer second, and a care provider a distant third.

Handling Conventional Doctors

Deep down, most doctors want to help people. They are higher than average in intelligence, and they have inquiring minds in spite of their training and the insurance and pharmaceutical companies. They are thus open to natural alternatives, but many doctors must be approached in a way that appeals to their technical knowledge and position in society.

My advice is that you read everything you can find on your child's illness or health care problems and ask lots of questions about various treatment options, the mechanisms of the illness, and the long-term prognoses associated with different options. But don't tell the doctor what you think your child has or what the treatment should be. If you do, it threatens the doctor's position of authority, making it far more unlikely that he or she will consider alternatives.

The best approach is to let the doctor feel in control but show that you have done your research, thereby giving the doctor a definite feeling of dealing with a partner. When they encounter an intelligent person who asks insightful questions, showing some understanding of medical terms, many doctors are willing to answer questions and discuss options. Most doctors will tell you that they learn a great deal more about medicine from their patients than they ever learned in medical school or from textbooks.

You are responsible for your child's life and health care. If your pediatrician or family doctor won't listen to your questions and won't discuss treatments in any detail despite repetitive queries on your part, then find another doctor. After all, it's your child, your peace of mind, your time, and your money that are at stake.

The Purpose of Complementary Medicine

The purpose of complementary medicine is not to replace traditional medical practices, but to supplement them or make them work better. While not considered standard by conservative authorities, these treatments are nevertheless practiced by licensed medical physicians who find them to be safe and effective, especially in patients who have not responded to conventional medical treatments. The prestigious U.S. National Institutes of Health in Bethesda, Maryland, has established a section to study complementary approaches to medical practice. The interest in complementary medicine is certainly spreading to areas of broad influence and the mainstream.

The real losers if alternative therapies are not judged scientifically or reasonably are the thousands of patients who have been helped after conventional allergy procedures had failed.

Appendix I:
Sources of Common Food Allergens

Foods and Products That Contain Corn

ale
aspirin
bacon
baking mixes: biscuits, donuts, pancake mixes, pie crusts
baking powder
batters for frying fish, poultry, meat
bee pollen
beers
beets, canned
beverages, carbonated
bleached white flours
bourbon and other whiskeys
breads and pastries
burritos
cakes
candy
cereals
cheeses
chili
chop suey
chow mein
coffee, instant
cola drinks
confectioner's sugar
corn flakes
cough syrups
crackers

cream of soy
cream puffs
custards
dates
deep-fat frying mixes
dextrose
eggnog
enchiladas
fish, prepared and processed
flour, bleached
French dressing
fried foods
frosting
fructose
fruit juices
fruit pies
fruits: canned, frozen
frying fats
gelatin desserts
glucose products
graham crackers
grape juice
gravies
grits
gin
gums, chewing
hams: cured, tenderized
hominy
honey

ice cream
jams
jellies
ketchup
leavening agents: baking powders, yeasts
lemonade
liquors: ale, beer, gin, whiskey
margarine
meats: bacon, bologna, ham, luncheon meats, sausages, wieners
MSG
noodles
pastries: cakes, cupcakes
peanut butter
peas, canned
pickles
pies, cream
pork and beans
powdered sugar
preserves
puddings and custards
ravioli
root beer
salad dressings
sandwich spreads
sauces: meat, fish, sundae

sausages
seasoning salt
sherbets
soft drinks
soups:
    creamed,
    vegetable
soybean milk

spaghetti
string beans: canned,
    frozen
sugar: powdered
syrups, commercially
    prepared
tamales
tea, instant

vegetables: canned,
    creamed, frozen
vinegar, distilled
whiskeys: American
    brandies, bourbon,
    Scotch
wines: fortified,
    sparkling

Food Products That Contain Eggs

angel food cake
baking powder
batters for deep
    frying
Bavarian cream
bouillon
breads
cakes
candies
cocoa drinks
consommé
cookies
cream pies
croquettes
custards
dessert powders
donuts
dumplings
egg in any form:
    creamed, deviled,
    dried, powdered,

fried, hard-boiled,
    poached
French toast
fritters
frostings
glazed rolls
griddle cakes
hamburger
    mix
hollandaise
    sauce
ice cream
icings
macaroni
macaroons
marshmallows
meat jellies
meat loaf
meringues
muffins
noodles

omelets
pancakes
patties
pie fillings
pretzels
puddings
root beer
salad dressings
sauces
sausages
sherbets
soufflés
soups
spaghetti
sponge cakes
tartar sauce
timbales
waffle mixes
waffles
whips
wines

Food Products That Contain Milk or Casein

"au gratin" foods
baker's bread
baking powder
    biscuits
Bavarian cream
bologna
butter
buttermilk

butter sauces
cakes
candies
cheese of all types
chocolate or cocoa
chowders
cream
cream sauces

curd
custards
donuts
flour mixes
food fried in butter:
    fish, poultry, beef,
    pork
fritters

gravies
hamburgers
hotcakes
ice cream
malted milk
mashed potatoes
meat, commercially
  prepared: poultry,
  fish, luncheon meats
milk in any form:
  condensed, dried,
  evaporated, malted,
  powdered
oleomargarine

omelets
pie crusts
pizza
popcorn
popovers
puddings
salad dressings
sausage, cooked
scrambled and scal-
  loped dishes
sherbets
soda crackers
some "non-dairy"
  products, such as

soy milk or
  soy cheeses
soufflés
soups: milk or
  creamed
Spanish cream
spumoni
waffles
whey
whipped-cream
  toppings
white sauce
yogurt

Dairy Substitutions

The following may be substituted for dairy products:

amazake (rice nectar
  drink)
fresh-fruit sorbets
frozen or fresh-fruit
  smoothies
frozen rice desserts
frozen tofu desserts

fruit ice cubes
juice popsicles
nut milk (almond
  milk, cashew milk)
rice-grain beverages
soy cheese (products
  that contain

casein or caseinate,
  which are milk
  proteins, should
  be avoided)
soy milk
tofu sour cream

Soy-Containing Products

The following foods usually contain soy, which is a ubiquitous
food used as a flour, oil, milk, and nut alternative:

bean curd
boxed breakfast
  cereals
butter substitutes
candies
caramels
chocolate
coffee substitutes
cold cuts
emulsifiers
hamburger

hamburger extender
hot dogs
ice cream
lecithin
lecithin spread
macaroni
margarine
mayonnaise
meat loaf
miso
nut candies

processed cheese
protein drinks
roasted soy nuts
  (sometimes used in
  place of peanuts)
salad dressings
sausages
sherbet
some breads, rolls,
  cakes, pastries,
  packaged mixes

soybean sprouts
soy flakes
soy grits
soy milk
soy noodles

soy sauce
spaghetti
tamari
tempeh
tofu

TVP (textured vege-
 table protein)
vegetable oils (may
 contain soy oil)
Worcestershire sauce

Food Products That Contain Wheat

ale, beer
au gratin potatoes
baking powder
bologna
bouillon cubes
bran flakes
bread and crackers
cakes
candy bars
canned/instant soup
casseroles
chili con carne
chocolate
cocomalt
cold cuts
cookies
corn flakes
cornmeal muffins
crackers
cream soups
creamed potatoes
croquettes
donuts
dumplings
farina
fats used in frying
fish patties
fish rolled in flour

floured, fried
 vegetables
fowl rolled in flour
frankfurters/wieners
frozen pies
gin
graham crackers
graham flour
gravies
griddle cakes
hamburger mix
hamburgers
hotcakes
ice cream
ice cream cones
liverwurst
macaroni mix
malt products
malted cereals
malted milk
matzos
mayonnaise
meat dishes, cooked
meat loaf
meats rolled in flour
MSG
muffins
noodles

pancake mixes
pies
pretzels
puddings
puffed wheat
pumpernickel
 bread
rolls
rye bread
salad dressing
sausage, cooked
scalloped potatoes
sherbets
shredded wheat
soufflés
soy bread
spaghetti
stuffing
sweet rolls
Swiss steak
synthetic pepper
timbales
vitamin E supple-
 ments
whiskey
white bread
whole wheat flour
zwieback

Appendix II: Diets and Food Components

Rotation Diet (also called Rotary Diversified Diet)

A four-day rotation diet is set up to prevent an individual from eating the same food more than once every four days. This prevents the development of new allergies due to overexposure to a particular food. A rotation diet also can control or reduce the impact of pre-existing food allergies. It is based on the principle that the less frequently one eats a certain food, such as wheat, the less likely it is that the food will become a new allergen. If the food is already a mild allergen, the rotation diet can prevent it from becoming a stronger allergen. Foods to which an individual has developed strong allergies are to be eliminated along with any foods from the same food family. Tolerated foods and foods in their food families are to be rotated every four days.

Rotation Diet

Day 1	Day 2	Day 3	Day 4
lean beef, veal, wild game, dairy	haddock, cod, mackerel, sole, snapper, salmon, herring, halibut, sardines	chicken, guinea hen, turkey, duck, eggs	clams, lobster, scallops
squash, pumpkin, zucchini, cucumber, sweet potatoes, water chestnuts	lettuce, endive, dandelion, cabbage, broccoli, turnips, radishes, cauliflower, kale mustard greens	all peas and beans, lentils, soy, leeks, alfalfa sprouts, carrots, celery, parsnips, parsley, asparagus, onions	potatoes, beets, tomatoes, corn, Swiss chard, peppers, eggplant

(continues)

Rotation Diet

Day 1	Day 2	Day 3	Day 4
peaches, figs, nectarines, dates, cherries, prunes, pineapple, melons, plums, apricots	bananas, grapes, raisins, blueberries, cranberries, persimmons, guavas	apples, pears, strawberries, raspberries, papayas, mangoes, rhubarb	oranges, lemons, grapefruit, tangerines, avocado, pomegranates
almonds, pumpkin seeds, macadamia nuts	pecans, walnuts, sunflower seeds	peanuts, cashews, soy nuts, pistachios	Brazil nuts, filberts, pine nuts, chestnuts
wheat, oats, rye, barley	quinoa, rice, tapioca	millet, buckwheat, arrowroot	corn, popcorn
date sugar, molasses	maple syrup, *stevia*	buckwheat honey	corn syrup
almond oil, canola oil	fish oil, sunflower oil	soy oil, peanut oil, sesame oil	olive oil, flax oil
black pepper, nutmeg, vanilla	sage, basil, rosemary, thyme, mustard, oregano, cloves	garlic, chives, ginger, turmeric, dill, fennel caraway, cumin, coriander	chili, cayenne, paprika, cinnamon, bay leaf, red pepper
rose hips	chamomile, blueberry, mint	parsley, alfalfa, sarsaparilla	juniper berry, comfrey, sassafras

Sample Elimination Diet

Eat only the foods listed; eat as much as you wish during the day, except for certain foods which may only be eaten on a four-day rotation basis as indicated below. The more varied the diet, the better for testing purposes.

Fruits

Pomegranates, pears, papaya, peaches, cherries, apricots, mangoes, plums, grapes, raisins, pineapple, fresh figs.

Vegetables

Cucumbers, zucchini, broccoli, bok choy, summer squash, crookneck squash, collard greens, celery, spinach, snow peas, chard, kale, cabbage, green beans, cauliflower, red and green leaf lettuce, sprouts, romaine lettuce, carrots, beets, parsley, watercress.

Starches

Sweet potatoes, spaghetti squash, yams, split peas, butternut squash, acorn squash, green peas, artichoke, buckwheat.

Meats and Fish

Lamb, duck, quail, venison, moose, cod, halibut, swordfish, shark, mackerel, herring.

Beverages

Avoid tap water; use distilled water, filtered water, or a pure bottled water. Fruit juices from allowable fruits only, diluted at least fifty percent. Use fresh juices rather than concentrates. Herbal teas are allowed: peppermint, rose hip, ginger root, ginseng. Beet, celery, cucumber, and carrot drink.

Oils

Cold-pressed flaxseed oil, olive and sunflower oils.

Salt

Sea salt or kelp powder.

Foods to Be Eaten Only Every Four Days

Apple, banana, melons, berries, chicken, turkey, rice, millet.

Gluten-Free, Dairy-Free Diet

Avoid the following foods, which contain gluten: wheat, rye, oats, barley, amaranth, triticale, spelt, and kamut.

Avoid all foods containing dairy products.

Upon arising: Any fruit of your choice. If no fresh fruit is available, four ounces or less of fruit juice mixed with an equal amount of water. Eat breakfast within twenty minutes of consuming this fruit or juice.

Breakfast: Eggs with olive oil and a raw or cooked vegetable. Water or herb tea.

Lunch: Vegetable or lentil/legume soup; chicken, turkey, or fish; salad with cooked vegetables, apple cider vinegar, and flaxseed oil.

Dinner: Same as lunch.

Bedtime: Portion of protein saved from dinner with salad or vegetable.

All through the day: Small snacks as frequently as desired, such as one to two teaspoons of mixed nuts and seeds or nut butter, vegetable juice, or diluted fruit juice. For "bread" add raw celery, broccoli, carrots, radishes, cucumbers, olives, lettuce, or cabbage.

Avoid:
- All sugars and honey, molasses, jelly, syrup, maltose, dextrose, fructose, and artificial sweeteners.
- Noodles, macaroni, spaghetti, wheat and wheat products (wheat germ, wheat germ oil).
- Regular bread, crackers, matzos, potato chips, and pretzels.
- Cakes, pastries, pie, candies, chewing gum, cashews, and chocolate.
- Cocoa, caffeinated drinks, and other sweet soft drinks.

Foods High in Potassium

In portions of $1/2$ cup, or $3 1/2$ ounces, or 100 grams. Most fruits and vegetables contain potassium, but these are some of the best sources:

almonds	773 mg	peanuts, roasted	701 mg
avocados	604 mg	pecans	603 mg
bananas	370 mg	pistachio nuts	972 mg
beef, cooked	370 mg	rabbit	368 mg
Brazil nuts	715 mg	rockfish	446 mg
chicken, cooked		salmon	361 mg
light meat	411 mg	sardines	590 mg
dark meat	321 mg	shad	377 mg
cod, cooked	407 mg	soy flour	1,660 mg
flounder	587 mg	squash, winter, baked	461 mg
filberts	704 mg	sweetbreads	433 mg
haddock	348 mg	tomato purée	426 mg
halibut	525 mg	turkey,	
liver, beef	380 mg	light meat	411 mg
liver, calf	453 mg	dark meat	398 mg
liver, pork	395 mg	veal	500 mg
milk, fresh	144 mg	walnuts	450 mg
milk, dried skim	1,725 mg	weakfish	465 mg

Sugar Content of Popular Foods

Food Item	Size of Portion	Teaspoons of Sugar
Beverages:		
cola drinks	6 oz.	$3^1/_2$
ginger ale	6 oz.	5
orange soda	8 oz.	5
root beer	10 oz.	$4^1/_2$
soda pop	8 oz.	5
sweet cider	1 cup	6
Cakes and cookies:		
angel food cake	4 oz.	7
applesauce cake	4 oz.	$5^1/_2$
banana cake	2 oz.	2
brownies (unfrosted)	$3/_4$ oz.	3
cheesecake	4 oz.	2
chocolate cake (plain)	4 oz.	6
chocolate cake (iced)	4 oz.	10
chocolate cookies	1	$1^1/_2$
chocolate eclair	1	7
coffeecake	4 oz.	$4^1/_2$
cream puff	1	2
cupcake (iced)	1	6
donut (plain)	1	3
donut (glazed)	1	6
fruit cake	4 oz.	5
gingersnaps	1	3
jelly roll	2 oz.	$2^1/_2$
macaroons	1	6
nut cookies	1	$1^1/_2$
oatmeal cookies	1	2
orange cake	4 oz.	4
pound cake	4 oz.	5
sponge cake	1 oz.	2
sugar cookies	1	$1^1/_2$

Sugar Content of Popular Foods

FOOD ITEM	SIZE OF PORTION	TEASPOONS OF SUGAR
Candies:		
butterscotch chew	1	1
chewing gum	1	$1/2$
chocolate bar	$1^1/_2$ oz.	$2^1/_2$
chocolate cream	1	2
chocolate mints	1	2
fudge	1 oz.	$4^1/_2$
gumdrop	1	2
hard candy	4 oz.	20
peanut brittle	1 oz.	$3^1/_2$
Canned fruits and juices:		
canned apricots	4 halves, 1 tablespoon syrup	$3^1/_2$
canned fruit juices	$1/2$ cup	2
canned peaches	2 halves, 1 tablespoon syrup	$3^1/_2$
fruit salad	$1/2$ cup	$3^1/_2$
fruit syrup	2 tablespoons	$2^1/_2$
stewed fruits	$1/2$ cup	2
Dairy products:		
ice cream	$1/3$ pint ($3^1/_2$ oz.)	$3^1/_2$
ice cream cone	1	$3^1/_2$
ice cream soda	1	5
ice cream sundae	1	7
malted milk shake	10 oz.	5
Desserts, miscellaneous:		
apple cobbler	$1/2$ cup	3
apple pie	1 slice (average)	7
apricot pie	1 slice	7
banana pudding	$1/2$ cup	2
berry pie	1 slice	10

(continues)

Sugar Content of Popular Foods

FOOD ITEM	SIZE OF PORTION	TEASPOONS OF SUGAR
berry tart	1 cup	10
blancmange	$1/2$ cup	5
blueberry cobbler	$1/2$ cup	3
bread pudding	$1/2$ cup	$1 1/2$
brown Betty	$1/2$ cup	3
butterscotch pie	1 slice	4
cherry pie	1 slice	10
chocolate pudding	$1/2$ cup	4
cornstarch pudding	$1/2$ cup	$2 1/2$
cream pie	1 slice	4
custard	$1/2$ cup	2
date pudding	$1/2$ cup	7
fig pudding	$1/2$ cup	7
French pastry	4 oz.	5
fruit gelatin	$1/2$ cup	$4 1/2$
lemon pie	1 slice	7
mincemeat pie	1 slice	4
peach pie	1 slice	7
plain pastry	4 oz.	3
plum pudding	$1/2$ cup	4
prune pie	1 slice	6
pumpkin pie	1 slice	5
rhubarb pie	1 slice	4
rice pudding	$1/2$ cup	5
sherbet	$1/2$ cup	9
tapioca pudding	$1/2$ cup	3

Syrups, sugars, and icings:

brown sugar	1 tablespoon	3
chocolate icing	1 oz.	5
chocolate sauce	1 tablespoon	$3 1/2$
corn syrup	1 tablespoon	3

Sugar Content of Popular Foods

Food Item	Size of Portion	Teaspoons of Sugar
honey	1 tablespoon	3
maple syrup	1 tablespoon	5
molasses	1 tablespoon	$3^1/_2$
white icing	1 oz.	5
Other:		
white bread	1 slice	$^1/_2$
corn flakes, frosted	$^1/_2$ cup	4–8
hamburger/ hot dog roll	1	3

Appendix III: Vitamin, Mineral, and Herb Suppliers

**Advanced Nutritional
Research**
One Washington St.
P.O. Box 807
Ellicottville, NY 14731
1-800-836-0644

Allergy Research Group
400 Preda St.
San Leandro, CA 94577
1-800-545-9960

**AMNI (Advanced
Medical Nutrition Inc.)**
2247 National Ave.
P.O. Box 5012
Hayward, CA 94540
1-800-437-8888

**BHI (Biological
Homeopathic
Industries, Inc.)**
11600 Cochiti SE
Albuquerque, NM 87123
1-800-621-7644

Bioquest Imports
1395 Marine Dr.
Box 27104
West Vancouver, BC V7T 2X8
CANADA
604-925-4728
Fax: 604-922-4649

**Bio-Therapeutics/
Phyto-Pharmica**
P.O. Box 1745
Green Bay, WI 54305
1-800-553-2370

**Biotics Research Corp.
Probiologic, Inc.**
14714 NE 87th St.
Redmond, WA 98052
1-800-678-8218

**J. R. Carlson
Laboratories, Inc.**
15 College Dr.
Arlington Hts., IL 60004-1985
1-800-323-4141

DaVinci Laboratories
20 New England Dr.
Essex Junction, VT 05453
1-800-325-1776

Dolisos America, Inc.
3014 Rigel Ave.
Las Vegas, NV 89102
1-800-365-4767

Douglas Laboratories
Wabash & Main
P.O. Box 8583
Pittsburgh, PA 15220
412-937-0122

Emerson Ecologics Inc.
436 Great Rd.
Acton, MA 01720
1-800-654-4432

**Enzyme Process
Laboratories, Inc.**
1 Commercial Ave.
Garden City, NY 11530
1-800-521-8669

For Your Health Pharmacy
13215 SE 240th St.
Kent, WA 98042
1-800-456-4325

**Greens Plus
Orange Peel Enterprises, Inc.**
730 14th St.
Vero Beach, FL 32960
1-800-643-1210 (U.S.);
1-800-387-4761 (Canada)

Jo Mar Laboratories
251 East Hacienda Ave.
Campbell, CA 95008
1-800-538-4545

Klabin Marketing
115 Central Park West
New York, NY 10023
212-877-3632
(in New York State);
1-800-933-9440 (elsewhere)

Klaire Laboratories
1573 W. Seminole St.
San Marcos, CA 92069
619-744-9680;
1-800-533-7255 (outside
California)

Life Extension Foundation
P.O. Box 229120
Hollywood, FL 33022-9120
305-966-4886;
1-800-841-LIFE

Murdock Pharmaceuticals
1400 Mountain Springs Park
Springville, UT 84663
1-800-962-8873

Natren
3105 Willow Lane
Westlake Village, CA 91361
1-800-992-3323;
1-800-992-9393 (in California)

**Nutraceutics Corp.
(DHEA Max)**
600 Fairway Dr., Suite 105
Deerfield Beach, FL 33441
1-800-391-0114

NutriPharm, Inc.
Birmingham, AL 35243
1-800-88-OMEGA
(800-886-6342)

Pathway Apothecary Pharmacy
5415 Cedar Lane
Bethesda, MD 20814
301-530-1112

Probiologic, Inc.
West Willows Technology
Center
14714 NE 87th St.
Redmond, WA 98052
1-800-678-8218

Professional Health Products
4307-49 St.
Innisfail, AB T4G 1P3
CANADA
1-800-661-1366

Progressive Laboratories, Inc.
1-800-527-9512

**Scandinavian Natural Health
and Beauty Products, Inc.**
13 North 7th St.
Perkasie, PA 18944
215-453-2505

Standard Homeopathic Co.
210 W. 131st St.
Box 61067
Los Angeles, CA 90061
213-321-4284

Supplements Plus
451 Church St.
Toronto, ON M4Y 2C5
CANADA
416-962-8369;
1-800-387-4761
Fax: 416-961-4033

Reliable information and sales
of nutritional, herbal, and
homeopathic remedies.

**Thorne Research
Products**
Sandpoint, ID 83864
1-800-228-1966

UAS Laboratories
9201 Penn Ave. South #10
Minneapolis, MN 55431
1-800-422-3371

**Vitamin Information Program
Hoffmann-La Roche Ltd.**
2455 Meadowpine Blvd.
Mississauga, ON L5N 6L7
CANADA
905-542-5615
Fax: 905-542-7130

Free literature and copies of
research studies on vitamins,
antioxidants for health professionals.

Appendix IV: Practitioner Referrals, Information, and Support Groups

Free Updates and New Information from Dr. Zoltan Rona

The author provides updates and new articles on nutritional medical topics free on the Internet. Dr. Rona's articles are available at the following web sites:

http://www.wwonline.com/rona/zpr
http://www.selene.com/healthlink/zpr.html
http://www.naturallink.com/homepages/zoltan_rona/index.html
http://www.yorku.ca/admin/wellness/articles.htm
http://www.allabouthealth.com/Current/Columns/RonaTOC.
   htm
http://www.infoserve.net/selene/healthlink/zpr.html

Referral Organizations

These organizations provide referrals, but you are responsible for verifying that a practitioner's training, experience, and level of expertise are appropriate for your specific needs.

American Association of Naturopathic Physicians
2366 Eastlake Avenue East, Suite 322
Seattle, WA 98102
206-323-7610
http://infinity.dorsai.org/Naturopathic.Physician

Send $5 for national directory with referrals to over 500 members who have completed postgraduate naturopathic medical education, including therapeutic nutrition, botanical medicine, counseling, homeopathy, and physical medicine.

American College for Advancement in Medicine (ACAM)
23121 Verdugo Drive, Suite 204
Laguna Hills, CA 92653
714-583-7666

American Holistic Medical Association
4101 Lake Boone Trail, Suite 201
Raleigh, NC 27607
919-787-5181

Send $8 for complete directory of 575 member M.D.s and Doctors of Osteopathy (D.O.s or osteopaths) with current unrestricted licenses.

Canadian Naturopathic Association
4174 Dundas St. W, Suite 304
Etobicoke, Ontario M8X 1X3
CANADA
President: Eugene Pontius, ND 604-992-5712
Executive Director: Heather MacFarland 416-233-1043
Fax: 416-233-2924

Foundation for Toxic-Free Dentistry
P.O. Box 608010
Orlando, FL 32860-8010
407-299-4149

Information and referrals to biologic dentists.

The General Council and Register of Naturopaths
Secretary: Mario Szewiel ND, DO, LicAc (Hons), MRN
Goswell House
2 Goswell Road
Somerset, England BA16 0JG
Tel: +44 1458 840072
Fax: +44 1458 840075
http://www.compulink.co.uk/~naturopathy/welcome.htm
gcrn_admin@naturopathy.compulink.co.uk

Holistic Dental Association
P.O. Box 5007
Durango, CO 81301

Offers referrals to 100 member dentists nationally who use complementary methods. Written requests only. Must enclose self-addressed, stamped envelope. Referrals are free but a donation is requested.

International Health Foundation, Inc.
Box 3494
Jackson, TN 38303

Provides international roster of physicians interested in candida-related disorders; helps children with repeated ear infections, hyperactivity, attention deficits, and related behavior and learning problems.

National College of Naturopathic Medicine
11231 Southeast Market St.
Portland, OR 97216
503-255-4860

For referrals to naturopathic doctors in your area.

National Institutes of Health

Office of Alternative Medicine
6120 Executive Boulevard
Rockville, MD 20092-9904
301-402-2466

Information Organizations

American Academy of Biological Dentistry
P.O. Box 856
Carmel Valley, CA 93924
408-659-5385
Fax: 408-659-2417

Promotes nontoxic diagnostic and therapeutic approaches to clinical dentistry.

American Academy of Environmental Medicine
P.O. Box 16106
Denver, CO 80216
303-622-9755

American Association of Naturopathic Physicians
P.O. Box 20386
Seattle, WA 98102
1-800-235-5800

American College of Nutrition
722 Robert E. Lee Drive
Wilmington, NC 28480
919-452-1222

Produces a journal and newsletter; provides lectures on nutrition research.

**American Holistic Medical Association and
American Holistic Nurses Association**
4101 Lake Boone Trail, Suite 201
Raleigh, NC 27607
1-800-878-3373; 919-787-5146

American Natural Hygiene Society
P.O. Box 30630
Tampa, FL 33630
813-855-6608

Aspartame Consumer Safety Network
P.O. Box 7806
Dallas, TX 75378
214-352-4268

Documentation of the hazards of aspartame consumption
and other information.

British Columbia Naturopathic Association
#204 - 2786 West 16th Ave.
Vancouver, BC V6K 3C4
CANADA
604-732-7070

**CFIDS Association (for information on the
chronic fatigue syndrome)**
P.O. Box 220398
Charlotte, NC 28222-0398
1-800-442-3437; 900-988-2343 (information line)
Fax: 704-365-9755

The largest organization for information on CFS and immune
dysfunction syndrome.

Consumer Health Organization of Canada
280 Sheppard Ave. E, #207
P.O. Box 248
Willowdale, Ontario M2N 5S9
CANADA
416-222-6517

DAMS (Dental Amalgam Mercury Syndrome)
725-9 Tramway Lane NE
Albuquerque, NM 87122
505-291-8239
Fax: 505-294-3339

Newsletter and other information dedicated to informing the public about the potential risks of mercury in dental amalgam fillings.

EDTA Chelation Lobby Association of B.C.
P.O. Box 67514, Station O
Vancouver, BC V5W 3T9
CANADA
604-327-3889

Environmental Dental Association
9974 Scripps Ranch Blvd., Suite 36
San Diego, CA 92131
619-586-1208
Fax: 619-693-0724

Educational, research, referral, and other resources for nontoxic dentistry.

The Food Allergy Network
10400 Eaton Place, Suite 107
Fairfax, VA 22030-2208
703-691-3179
Fax: 703-691-2713

Nonprofit organization that puts out a newsletter ($24.00/yr U.S.$) on food allergies; covers allergy-related subjects such as eczema, allergen-free recipes, drug updates, and news updates and carries a dietitian's column. They also sell a number of reasonably priced booklets and cards with information on how to cope with schools, anaphylaxis (potentially lethal allergic reactions), and how to read food labels so as to avoid allergens (e.g., soy products go by many names in packaging). Sample newsletter and information sent on request.

Great Lakes Association of Clinical Medicine (GLACM)
70 West Huron Street
Chicago, IL 60610
Contact: Mr. Jack Hank, executive director
312-266-7246

Nonprofit corporation whose membership includes holistic physicians from the United States and other countries. Regular meetings are held to update members on latest developments in medical practice and patient care. Seminars presented on a regular basis.

Herb Research Foundation
1007 Pearl St., Suite 200
Boulder, CO 80302
303-449-2265

Listing of practitioners knowledgeable about herbs. Members receive *HERBALGRAM,* a quarterly which presents research reviews from the scientific literature and follows legal issues, market trends, and media coverage of herbs.

The ME (Chronic Fatigue Syndrome) Association of Canada
400 - 246 Queen St.
Ottawa, Ontario K1P 5E4
CANADA
613-563-1565
Fax: 613-567-0614

National Organization for Rare Disorders (NORD)
P.O. Box 8923
New Fairfield, CT 06812
203-746-6518

Nightingale Research Foundation
383 Danforth Ave.
Ottawa, Ontario K2A 0E1
CANADA
613-728-9643
Fax: 613-729-0825

Information and support groups for chronic fatigue syndrome/ ME.

World Research Foundation
15300 Ventura Blvd., Suite 405
Sherman Oaks, CA 91403
818-907-5483
Fax: 818-907-6044

Information on therapies inside and outside mainstream medicine for any health condition.

Periodicals

Alive
Canadian Journal of Health and Nutrition
Box 80055
Burnaby, BC V5H 3X1
CANADA
604-438-1919
Fax: 604-435-4888

Mail and messages received here for Dr. Z. Rona, *Alive* Advisor.

Free World News
Paul Coulbeck, Publisher and Editor-in-Chief
#1010-5334 Yonge Street
Willowdale, Ontario M2N 6V1
CANADA
416-590-9586, ext. 167
e-mail: free@inforamp.net
http://www.inforamp.net/~free/

The Townsend Letter for Doctors
911 Tyler St.
Port Townsend, WA 98368-6541

Monthly newsletter for natural health care practitioners; highly recommended for its political and editorial content.

Educational Institutions

Alive Academy of Nutrition
7436 Fraser Park Dr.
Burnaby, BC V5J 5B9
CANADA
604-435-1919
Fax: 604-435-4888

Home study nutrition course and other educational opportunities.

Bastyr College of Naturopathic Medicine
144 NE 54th St.
Seattle, WA 98105
206-523-9585

Courses and training in naturopathic medicine.

Canadian College of Naturopathic Medicine
60 Berl Avenue
Etobicoke, Ontario M8Y 3C7
CANADA
416-251-5261

Offers a diploma program in naturopathic medicine.

National College of Naturopathic Medicine
11231 SE Market Street
Portland, OR 97216
503-255-4860
Clinic: 503-255-7355

Southwest College of Naturopathic Medicine
6535 E. Osborn Rd., Suite 703
Scottsdale, AZ 85251
602-990-7424

Offers a degree program in naturopathic medicine.

Vaccination Information

Association for Vaccine Damaged Children
Mary James
67 Shier
Winnipeg, Manitoba R3R 2I12
CANADA
204-895-9192

Or contact Leona Rew
22 Malone St.
Winnipeg, Manitoba R3R 1L4
CANADA
204-895-4015

Information on the damaging effects of vaccinations, book lists, etc.

My Health, My Rights
2309 Horton St.
Ottawa, Ontario, K1G 3E7
CANADA
819-684-3060
Fax: 819-684-6351

This group deals with issues regarding freedom of choice in health care in Canada.

National Health Federation
P.O. Box 688
Monrovia, CA 91017
818-357-2181
Fax: 818-303-0642

$25.00 vaccine packet, includes two books.

National Vaccine Information Center (DPT/NVIC)
512 W. Maple Ave., Suite 206
Vienna, VA 22180
1-800-909-SHOT(7468); 703-938-0342
Fax: 703-938-5768
$25.00 (U.S.$) membership

Bulletins, lobbying, resources, books, etc.; information on vaccines and the prevention of vaccine damage.

Vaccine Information and Awareness (VIA)
c/o Karin Schumacher
P.O. Box 203482
Austin, TX 78720
512-832-4176
Fax: 512-873-8771
Email: via@eden.com

VIA empowers parents to question, challenge, investigate, research, and become more informed and aware about the risks that exist with vaccines. The major philosophy of this group is to ensure that freedom of choice is not taken away from each parent. The decision to vaccinate is one that should and must be made by the parent alone. To this end VIA:

- Maintains a mailing list to inform people about current events, medical findings and research, legal events, and other facts regarding vaccinations.
- Manages the National Vaccine Information Center (NVIC) and Vaccine Information and Awareness (VIA) Web sites.
- Works with state representatives to get legislation amended to include a philosophical exemption in addition to the existing religious and medical exemptions.
- Provides information and resources by mail, phone, email, newspaper, radio, and television for parents who have questions or concerns about vaccine safety and efficacy.
- Holds monthly support group meetings.
- Works with civil liberty organizations to ensure parents the right to freedom of choice where vaccines are concerned.
- Contacts celebrities and high-profile personalities to help promote parents' right to make a nonmandated, informed decision.
- Investigates and researches medical and scientific claims on vaccine safety and efficacy.

Variance
814 Shaw St.
Toronto, Ontario M6G 3M1
CANADA
416-534-1477

A Canadian group concerned with similar issues as VIA.

Glossary

Acupuncture: a Chinese system of medicine which involves the use of needles or another form of stimulation of certain points of the body that improve the flow of vital energy *(Qi)* along pathways called meridians. (Meridians are distinct from the anatomical nervous system network.) Needles, heat, laser, or electrical stimuli can be applied to the acupuncture points. The Chinese use acupuncture combined with herbs to treat all disease conditions.

Allergen: a substance, which can be a food, chemical, or environmental particle, which is capable of producing an allergic response.

Allergy: term used to describe an abnormal reaction to an allergen which is generally well tolerated by healthy individuals.

Antigen: any molecule that induces the formation of antibodies (e.g., a virus, bacteria, or even one's own tissue).

Antioxidant: molecule capable of neutralizing free radicals, which are highly reactive and destructive molecules. It is theorized that antioxidants can prevent, slow, or reverse organ degeneration, aging, and disease. The best-known and most-studied antioxidants are vitamins C, and E, selenium, and beta carotene.

Autoimmune disease: disease caused by a defect in the immune system which causes the body's normal tolerance of its own tissues to disappear. Antibodies may start attacking cells, tissues, and organs, leading to such conditions as lupus, rheumatoid arthritis, diabetes, multiple sclerosis, and dozens of other diseases.

Environmental medicine: term used for the medical specialty which treats allergic illnesses; especially known for treatment of multiple chemical sensitivity and chronic fatigue syndrome. Formerly referred to as clinical ecology, environmental medicine uses primarily natural techniques of diagnosis and treatment. These may include nutritional medicine, special diets, electroacupuncture, herbology, homeopathy, desensitization therapies, and the treatment of electric field imbalances.

Free radical: a molecule which contains an odd number of electrons, resulting in an unoccupied bond, which makes the molecule highly reactive (it seeks to "react" in order to complete the bond) and potentially destructive to cells, tissues, and organs.

Holistic medicine: a system of health care which fosters a cooperative relationship among all those involved, leading toward optimal attainment of the physical, mental, emotional, social, and spiritual aspects of health. It emphasizes the need to look at the whole person, including analysis of physical, nutritional, environmental, emotional, social, spiritual, and lifestyle values. It encompasses all modalities of diagnosis and treatment, including drugs and surgery if no safe alternative exists. Holistic medicine focuses on education and responsibility for personal efforts to achieve balance and well-being.

Homeopathy: a practice based on the principle of "like cures like," originated by physician and researcher Samuel Hahnemann two hundred years ago. These dilute remedies are gentle and powerful and can affect emotions and physical states without significant side effects.

Hydrotherapy: a therapy that uses the healing power of hot and cold water to promote circulation, improve bowel and immune function, relieve headaches, and treat acute infections. Using ice and heat for an injury is a form of hydrotherapy.

Immunoglobulins (IgA, D, G, M, E): a group of glycoproteins known as antibodies, present in the serum and tissue fluids of all mammals. They are produced by plasma cells and are integral to the adaptive immune response. There are five different classes of immunoglobulin molecules.

In vitro: research carried on outside the organism in glass or in another receptacle.

In vivo: research carried out in a living organism.

Lipids: fatty substances including fatty acids, fats, and soaps.

Lymphocytes: cells of the immune system that are responsible for the adaptive immune response. B-cell lymphocytes are produced in the bone marrow and make antibodies. T-cell lymphocytes are produced in the thymus and are divided into different subsets based on their function within the immune system.

Naturopathic doctors (NDs): primary health care providers who use therapies that are almost exclusively natural and nontoxic, such as clinical nutrition, homeopathy, botanical (herbal) medicine, hydrotherapy, physical medicine, and lifestyle counseling. Modern naturopathic medicine is based on accredited educational institutions, professional licensing by a growing number of states, rigorous national standards of practice, peer review, and an ongoing commitment to state-of-the-art scientific research. Naturopathic practice includes the following diagnostic and treatment modalities: all methods of clinical and laboratory diagnostic testing, including diagnostic radiology and other imaging techniques; nutritional medicine, dietetics, and therapeutic fasting; medicines of mineral, animal, and botanical origin; hygiene and public health measures; homeopathy; acupuncture; Chinese medicine; psychotherapy and counseling; minor surgery and naturopathic obstetrics (natural childbirth); naturopathic physical medicine, including naturopathic manipulative therapies; hydrotherapy, heat, cold, ultrasound, and therapeutic exercise. Naturopathic practice excludes major surgery and the use of most synthetic drugs.

Peptides: a chain of two(di-), three (tri-), or more (poly-) amino acids.

T-cell: an immune cell produced in the thymus gland. Subsets of T-cells include T-helper, T-suppressor, and T-killer cells. T-cells become activated upon exposure to antigens.

Tincture: a liquid solution made by soaking an herb for several hours or days (depending upon the type of herb) in a mixture of solvents containing alcohol and water.

Traditional Chinese medicine (TCM): a system of natural healing which makes heavy use of acupuncture. By inserting sterile disposable needles into points on the body along the meridian channels, it regulates the *Qi* (energy) in the body in order to treat disease. The use of Chinese herbs and herbal formulas is another important part of TCM. TCM involves a complete theory for making a diagnosis and developing a treatment plan. For many kinds of pain, acupuncture should be the first choice, such as for joint pain (shoulder, elbow, wrist, hip, knee, ankle, and small joints), the pain after surgery, *herpes zoster*, phantom limb pain, sciatica, arthritis, migraine, etc.

Further Reading

Braly, James, M.D. *Dr. Braly's Food Allergy and Nutrition Revolution.* New Canaan, CT: Keats Publishing, Inc., 1992.

Braverman, Eric R. *The Healing Nutrients Within.* New Canaan, CT: Keats Publishing, Inc., 1987.

Buttram, H. E. *The Dangers of Immunization.* Richlandtown, PA: The Humanitarian Publishing Company, 1979. (P.O. Box 193, Richlandtown, PA 18955-0193; 1-800-282-0677.)

Buttram, H. F., and J. C. Hoffman. *Vaccination and Immune Malfunction.* Richlandtown, PA: The Humanitarian Publishing Company, 1982. (P.O. Box 193, Richlandtown, PA 18955-0193; 1-800-282-0677.)

Conners, C. Keith. *Feeding the Brain: How Foods Affect Children.* New York: Plenum, 1989.

Coulter, Harris L. *Vaccination, Social Violence, and Criminality: The Medical Assault on the American Brain.* Berkeley, CA: North Atlantic Books, 1990. (510-644-2116; fax: 510-652-4336.)

Crook, William G., M.D. *Solving the Puzzle of Your Hard-to-Raise Child.* Jackson, TN: Professional Books, 1987.

Crook, William G., M.D. *The Yeast Connection Handbook.* Jackson, TN: Professional Books, 1996.

Ford, Norman D. *18 Natural Ways to Beat Chronic Tiredness.* New Canaan, CT: Keats Publishing, Inc., 1993.

Freeman, John M. *The Epilepsy Diet Treatment: An Introduction to the Ketogenic Diet.* New York: Demos Publications, 1994.

Gelberg, Kitty H., Ph.D., M.P.H., et al. "Fluoride Exposure and Childhood Osteosarcoma: A Case-Control Study," *American Journal of Public Health*, 85(12) (December, 1995): 1678–1683.

Heimlich, Jane. *What Your Doctor Won't Tell You.* New York: Harper Collins, 1990.

Moore, Neecie. *Bountiful Health, Boundless Energy, Brilliant Youth: The Facts About DHEA.* Dallas: Charis Publishing Co., Inc., 1994.

Murray, Michael T. *Natural Alternatives to Over-the-Counter and Prescription Drugs.* New York: William Morrow and Company, Inc., 1994.

Rapp, Doris J., M.D. *Allergies and the Hyperactive Child.* New York: Cornerstone Library (Simon & Schuster), 1979.

Rapp, Doris J., M.D. *Allergies and Your Family.* New York: Sterling Publishing, 1980.

Rona, Zoltan P., M.D. *The Joy of Health.* Toronto, Canada: Hounslow Press, 1991.

Rona, Zoltan P., M.D. *Return to the Joy of Health.* Vancouver, Canada: Alive Books, 1995.

Zukin, Jane. *Raising Your Child Without Milk: Reassuring Advice and Recipes for Parents of Lactose-Intolerant and Milk-Allergic Children.* Rocklin, CA: Prima Publishing, 1996.

Index

A

Ace-K, 43
Acesulfame-K, 43
Achlorhydria, 58
Acid-suppressing drugs, 20
ACS, *see* American Cancer
  Society
Acyclovir, 93
ADA, *see* American Dental
  Association; American
  Diabetes Association
ADD, *see* Attention deficit
  disorder
Addictions, 146–147
Adrenal insufficiency, 38–39
Air contamination, 16–17
Alcoholism, 13
Algae, blue-green, 120
Allergic rhinitis, 144–146
  symptoms, 144
  treatment, 145–146
Allergies
  aspirin, 64
  chemical, *see* Chemical
    allergies
  conventional treatment, 4–5
  definition, 3
  digestion and, 17–26
  environmental factors, 5,
    13–16
  food, *see* Food allergies
  incidence, 98

LD and, 184–185
  medications for, prob-
    lems, 185
  related illnesses, 136, 144–146
  salicylates, 64
Allergy tests, 55–57
  CDSA, 57–59
  environmental sensitivity,
    49–50
  food sensitivity, 49–50
Aloe vera
  for autoimmune disease, 140
Alpha-tocopherol
  as aspirin alternative, 105
  for autoimmune diseases,
    143–144
  benefits, 130
  iron and, effects, 77
Alternative medicine
  conventional doctors and,
    202–204
AMA, *see* American Medical
  Association
Amazake, 41–42
American Academy of Head,
  Neck, and Facial Pain, 35
American Cancer Society, 201
American Dental Associa-
  tion, 35
American Diabetes
  Association, 44–45

World Health Organization,
88, 136
Wright, Dr. Jonathan, 191

X

Xenobiotics, 131–132

Y

Yucca, 106

Z

Zinc
ADD and, 178
benefits, 130–131
calcium and, effects, 77
for chronic coughs, 92
nephrotic syndrome
and, 200
rich foods, 196
Zinc gluconate lozenges, 92